TEST ITEM FILE

KATHERINE M. KITZMANN
THOMAS F. OLTMANNS
ROBERT E. EMERY

ABNORMAL PSYCHOLOGY

THOMAS F. OLTMANNS

ROBERT E. EMERY

PRENTICE HALL, *Englewood Cliffs, New Jersey 07632*

©1995 by PRENTICE-HALL, INC.
A Simon and Schuster Company
Englewood Cliffs, New Jersey 07632

10 9 8 7 6 5 4 3 2 1

ISBN 0-13-148784-1
Printed in the United States of America

Table of Contents

Note to the Instructor

We created this testbank for use with the text <u>Abnormal Psychology</u>, by Thomas F. Oltmanns and Robert E. Emery. It represents a collaborative effort, in which the text authors were actively involved in developing test items that would reflect the text's emphasis on the systems approach to understanding abnormal psychology. We are enthusiastic about the final product, which we believe will be a useful resource for instructors.

For each chapter of the textbook, the testbank includes about 75 multiple choice questions, about 20 true-false questions, and about 5 essay or short answer questions.

After each question, the correct answer is listed along with a brief description of the type of question, its difficulty level, the kind of knowledge assessed, and the page number where the correct answer can be found in the text. Following are the abbreviations used:

<u>Type of question</u>:   **MC** (multiple choice)
          TF (true-false)
          ES (essay or short answer)

<u>Difficulty level</u>:   **Easy**
         Mod (moderate)
         Diff (difficult)

<u>Kind of knowledge assessed</u>: **f** (factual)
             c (conceptual)
             a (applied)

These test items have also been incorporated into the **Prentice Hall Test Manager**, a computerized testbank that is available for IBM PCs and compatibles. This test-generating software is user-friendly. It allows the instructor to select and arrange a subset of items and to print them quickly and easily in test form. Instructors can also add their own questions to the computerized testbank or customize those provided. It is an excellent system that can save considerable time and effort in constructing tests. To obtain a computerized version of the testbank, contact Prentice Hall directly (1-800-526-0485), or talk to your local sales representative.

-Katherine M. Kitzmann
-Thomas F. Oltmanns
-Robert E. Emery

Chapter 1
Examples and Definitions of Abnormal Behavior

Multiple Choice Questions

1.1: The "scientist-practitioner" model refers to:

    a) a training approach that integrates science and professional practice
    b) a system of research methods in abnormal psychology
    c) a clinician who supervises student therapists
    d) the use of psychiatric medications developed in the laboratory

MC/Easy
Pg:2
kind:f
Ans:(a)

1.2: Psychology is best described as:

    a) the treatment of mental disorders
    b) the scientific study of behavior and mental processes
    c) a philosophy of mind
    d) the scientific study of personality

MC/Easy
Pg:2
kind:f
Ans:(b)

1.3: Abnormal psychology is best described as:

    a) the treatment of mental disorders
    b) a personality trait
    c) a form of comparative psychology
    d) the application of psychological science to the study of mental disorders

MC/Easy
Pg:2
kind:f
Ans:(d)

1.4: According to the Epidemiologic Catchment Area (ECA) study, during a 12-month period, what percentage of Americans can be expected to exhibit active symptoms of at least 1 mental disorder?

    a) 1 in 3   b) 1 in 5
    c) 1 in 10   d) 1 in 20

MC/Diff
Pg:2
kind:f
Ans:(b)

1.5: According to the Epidemiologic Catchment Area (ECA) study, what percentage of Americans can be expected to experience at least one kind of mental disorder at some point during their lives?

    a) 1 in 3   b) 1 in 5
    c) 1 in 10   d) 1 in 20

MC/Diff
Pg:2
kind:f
Ans:(a)

1.6: Clinical psychology is a discipline that:

    a) is a branch of medicine concerned with treatment of mental disorders
    b) applies psychological science to the treatment of mental disorders
    c) focuses on neurological research
    d) focuses on the use of medication to treat mental disorder

MC/Easy
Pg:3
kind:f
Ans:(b)

1.7: Abraham Lincoln suffered from:

    a) schizophrenia   b) alcoholism
    c) depression   d) phobias

MC/Mod
Pg:3
kind:f
Ans:(c)

1.8: Psychiatrists have earned which degree?

    a) M.D.   b) Ph.D.
    c) Psy.D.   d) M.A.

MC/Easy
Pg:3
kind:f
Ans:(a)

1.9: Severe disruptions of verbal communication seen in psychotic disorders are called disorganized speech, also known as:

    a) delusions
    b) hallucinations
    c) formal thought disorder
    d) idiosyncratic symptomatology

MC/Mod
Pg:4
kind:f
Ans:(c)

1.10: Two landmark legal cases in the 1970s, Blue Shield of Virginia v. McCready, and Wyatt v. Stickney, found that licensed clinical psychologists:

    a) could treat patients without supervision by psychiatrists
    b) could practice psychoanalysis
    c) could not be reimbursed by insurance companies for services that could be provided by an M.D.
    d) had to purchase malpractice insurance in order to be licensed

MC/Mod
Pg:4
kind:f
Ans:(a)

1.11: Brian feels spiders crawling over his body, but no spiders are there. Brian is experiencing:

    a) a delusion
    b) formal thought disorder
    c) disorganized thinking
    d) an hallucination

MC/Mod
Pg:4
kind:a
Ans:(d)

1.12: Which of the following is true about the mental health professions (such as clinical psychology, psychiatry, and clinical social work)?

    a) only clinical psychologists are trained to conduct therapy
    b) the boundaries between professions change in response to economic and legal pressures
    c) only psychiatrists are licensed by state boards of examiners
    d) there is very little overlap in what clinical psychologists, psychiatrists, and clinical social workers do

MC/Mod
Pg:4
kind:c
Ans:(b)

1.13: The distinguishing characteristic of psychosis is:

    a) behavior that is disruptive to the community
    b) the need for medication
    c) symptoms secondary to head injury
    d) loss of contact with reality

MC/Mod
Pg:4
kind:f
Ans:(d)

1.14: A delusion is:

    a) an idiosyncratic belief not held by other members of society
    b) a perceptual experience in the absence of external stimulation
    c) formal thought disorder
    d) disorganized verbal communication

MC/Easy
Pg:4
kind:f
Ans:(a)

1.15: Which is an example of formal thought disorder?

    a) "I believe my television is transmitting messages from Mars."
    b) "I like reading the paper, but it's Tuesday and my cat has fleas."
    c) "I hear voices but my family says they don't hear anything."
    d) "I cannot remember details from one moment to the next."

MC/Mod
Pg:4
kind:a
Ans:(b)

1.16: Celia believes that each time an important public figure dies, one of the fish in her pond dies also. Her neighbors have tried to explain to her the absurdity of this idea, but she is rigid in her insistence. Celia may be experiencing:

   a) an hallucination
   b) a delusion
   c) formal thought disorder
   d) idiosyncratic symptomatology

1.17: Psychopathology is:

   a) a general term describing abnormal behavior
   b) a specific type of psychosis
   c) a severe form of mental illness
   d) a form of deviance often involving crime

1.18: A psychopathologist:

   a) does autopsies on suicide victims
   b) is a psychiatric patient
   c) studies abnormal behavior
   d) generally looks for biological causes of psychosis

1.19: Psychopathology is defined in terms of:

   a) inferred biological causes
   b) observations of behavior and descriptions of personal experience
   c) responses to psychological tests
   d) statistical frequency

1.20: Mental disorders are typically defined in terms of:

   a) one distinguishing symptom
   b) statistical rarity
   c) the individual being out of touch with reality
   d) a set of characteristic features

1.21: A syndrome is:

    a) a biologically-based mental illness
    b) a group of symptoms that usually appear
       together
    c) a condition with no official diagnosis
    d) the essential symptom, sufficient to make a
       diagnosis

MC/Easy
Pg:7
kind:f
Ans:(b)

1.22: Beth shows delusional thinking and hallucinations.
Bob shows hallucinations and formal thought
disorder. According to DSM-IV:

    a) they would be given different diagnoses
    b) they could both be classified as schizophrenic
    c) they probably have different etiologies
    d) they should get different treatments

MC/Diff
Pg:8
kind:a
Ans:(b)

1.23: People given a specific diagnosis (for example,
Major Depression):

    a) all show the same set of symptoms
    b) all have the same etiology
    c) would be given the same diagnosis in any
      culture
    d) show some of the same symptoms

MC/Mod
Pg:8
kind:c
Ans:(d)

1.24: The Diagnostic and Statistical Manual of Mental
Disorders, 4th Edition (DSM-IV) is published by:

    a) The American Psychological Association
    b) The World Health Organization
    c) The American Psychiatric Association
    d) The National Institutes of Mental Health

MC/Mod
Pg:9
kind:f
Ans:(c)

1.25: The definition of abnormal behavior in the DSM-IV
places primary emphasis on:

    a) biological disadvantage, e.g. in terms of
      reproduction
    b) personal distress or impairment in social
      functioning
    c) statistical rarity
    d) known biological etiology

MC/Diff
Pg:9
kind:c
Ans:(b)

1.26: The official criteria for the diagnosis of mental disorders are listed in:

MC/Easy
Pg:9
kind:f
Ans:(d)

a) American Psychiatric Association Guidelines for Diagnosis
b) Physicians Desk Reference
c) Diagnosis of Syndromes of Mental Illness
d) Diagnostic and Statistical Manual of Mental Disorders

1.27: Definitions of mental illness in the DSM-IV:

MC/Mod
Pg:10
kind:c
Ans:(d)

a) consider only behaviors that would be considered abnormal in any culture
b) are not influenced by political or cultural factors
c) include deviant behaviors that are encouraged by certain religions
d) recognize that some behaviors are abnormal in one society but not in another

1.28: Olivia grew up in a society where mourners pull out their hair, go into an emotional frenzy, and begin speaking in tongues. On a visit to the U.S., she did these things in public when she heard that a relative had died. According to DSM-IV, her behavior would be considered:

MC/Diff
Pg:10
kind:a
Ans:(b)

a) not psychopathological, because it caused no disruption in social functioning
b) not psychopathological, because it is part of her culture
c) psychopathological, because of her personal distress
d) psychopathological, because it disrupted her social functioning

1.29: In response to criticism by outside political groups about the possible diagnosis of premenstrual dysphoric disorder, the DSM-IV committee:

MC/Diff
Pg:10
kind:c
Ans:(b)

a) eliminated the category
b) recommended further study
c) changed the name to premenstrual syndrome (PMS)
d) issued a statement about the need for scientific committees not to be influenced by political concerns

1.30: Which is true about the role of value judgments in   MC/Mod
       the development of diagnostic systems?   Pg:11
                                                              kind:c
       a) values are inherent in any attempt to define   Ans:(a)
          disease
       b) values have no place in the attempt to define
          disease
       c) diagnosis is completely determined by values
       d) values can be avoided with the use of
          scientific methods

1.31: The threshold model of classification represents a: MC/Mod
                                                              Pg:13
       a) combination of the categorical and dimensional   kind:c
          approaches   Ans:(a)
       b) categorical approach
       c) dimensional approach
       d) biologically-based system

1.32: The DSM-IV uses which approach to classification?   MC/Easy
                                                              Pg:14
       a) threshold   b) etiological   kind:f
       c) dimensional   d) categorical   Ans:(d)

1.33: Diagnosis using the DSM-IV classification system   MC/Mod
       involves: Pg:14
                                                              kind:c
       a) describing behavior on a continuum   Ans:(d)
       b) identifying the cause or etiology of behavior
       c) making numerical ratings, below or above a
          critical threshold
       d) assigning a person's behavior to a specific
          category of mental disorder

1.34: Among normal-weight college women in the community,   MC/Mod
       what percentage would meet the criteria for bulimia   Pg:14
       nervosa?   kind:f
                                                              Ans:(b)
       a) 1%   b) 4%
       c) 16%   d) 30%

1.35: Among normal-weight college women in the community,   MC/Mod
       what percentage have engaged in purging behaviors?   Pg:14
                                                              kind:f
       a) 1%   b) 4%   Ans:(c)
       c) 16%   d) 40%

7

1.36: Epidemiology is the study of:

    a) biological causes of diseases
    b) classification systems for diagnosis
    c) frequency and distribution of disorders
    d) quickly spreading diseases

MC/Easy
Pg:14
kind:f
Ans:(c)

1.37: Which is an example of something an epidemiologist would do?

    a) study chromosomes to find abnormal genes associated with alcoholism
    b) encourage people with the flu not to drink alcohol
    c) study rates of alcoholism in urban versus rural areas
    d) investigate the effects of alcoholism on the body's immune system

MC/Mod
Pg:14
kind:c
Ans:(c)

1.38: An epidemiologist studies rates of depression in a community over a one-year period. Her calculation of incidence will be based on the:

    a) total number of active cases on the day of calculation
    b) number of new cases that developed during that year
    c) proportion of people who had ever been depressed
    d) average time between diagnosis and cure

MC/Mod
Pg:14
kind:c
Ans:(b)

1.39: In a small rural community, 2 people have had anxiety disorders in the past but not now. Three people developed anxiety disorders four or five years ago, and all 3 of these people continue to have an anxiety disorder now. Which of the following is true about the rate of anxiety disorders in this community during the last 6 months?

    a) incidence = 3
    b) prevalence = 5
    c) prevalence = 3
    d) lifetime prevalence = 5

MC/Diff
Pg:14
kind:c
Ans:(c)

8

1.40: Prior to 1940, many people who were admitted to psychiatric hospitals showing signs of schizophrenia actually were suffering from pellagra, caused by a vitamin deficiency. Epidemiologists contributed to the correct diagnosis of these individuals because they:

    a) found that a commonality among new cases was poverty and poor diet
    b) examined blood samples and found a vitamin deficiency
    c) interviewed patients and asked about family history of schizophrenia
    d) introduced poor diets to normals to see if they developed symptoms of schizophrenia

1.41: The symptoms of pellagra, a disease caused by vitamin deficiency, most closely resemble those of:

    a) depression   b) schizophrenia
    c) anxiety   d) eating disorders

1.42: What percentage of bulimic patients are female?

    a) 30%   b) 50%
    c) 70%   d) more than 85%

1.43: Compared to working women, among university women the incidence of bulimia is:

    a) half as great   b) about the same
    c) 5 times higher   d) 10 times higher

1.44: Jane Murphy's anthropological study of 2 nonwestern cultures, the Inuit and the Yoruba, led her to conclude that:

    a) western and nonwestern cultures recognize similar patterns of behavior as being "crazy"
    b) the behavior patterns called "crazy" in western cultures are very different from those called "crazy" in nonwestern cultures
    c) the concept of "craziness" may be limited to western cultures
    d) nonwestern cultures view "crazy" behavior as part of spiritual healing

9

1.45: The large scale epidemiological study of
schizophrenia in 9 countries, sponsored by the
World Health Organization (WHO), found:

MC/Diff
Pg:15
kind:f
Ans:(d)

a) higher rates of schizophrenia in developed
(western) countries
b) higher rates of schizophrenia in developing
(nonwestern) countries
c) different rates of schizophrenia depending on
each culture
d) similar rates of schizophrenia in developed and
developing countries

1.46: In which group are rates of bulimia thought to be
increasing?

MC/Easy
Pg:15
kind:f
Ans:(a)

a) affluent African-American women
b) poor African-American women
c) affluent European-American women
d) poor European-American women

1.47: Which disorder is more common in men than in women?

MC/Easy
Pg:16
kind:f
Ans:(a)

a) antisocial personality disorder
b) anxiety
c) mania
d) schizophrenia

1.48: Which disorder is about equally common in men and
women?

MC/Easy
Pg:16
kind:f
Ans:(a)

a) mania
b) depression
c) alcoholism
d) antisocial personality disorder

1.49: Which disorder is more common in women than men?

MC/Easy
Pg:16
kind:f
Ans:(b)

a) alcoholism   b) depression
c) schizophrenia   d) mania

10

1.50: The Epidemiologic Catchment Area (ECA) study   MC/Diff
       finding that lifetime prevalence rates are usually   Pg:16
       much higher than prevalence rates for the last 12   kind:c
       months suggests that mental illness: Ans:(a)

       a) often involves periods of remission or complete
          recovery
       b) is for the most part a chronic or enduring
          condition
       c) is more common now than in the past
       d) is more common in the elderly

1.51: Etiology refers to: MC/Easy
                                                          Pg:16
       a) the study of rates of various diseases and   kind:f
          disorders   Ans:(d)
       b) a philosophy of classification and diagnosis
       c) the course of a disorder
       d) the causes of a disorder

1.52: A case study is: MC/Easy
                                                          Pg:19
       a) a large scale study identifying rates of a   kind:f
          disorder in a population   Ans:(d)
       b) a psychological evaluation for legal purposes
       c) an analysis of an individual's behavior when
          under confinement
       d) a detailed description and analysis of one
          person

1.53: The primary limitation of case studies is that they: MC/Diff
                                                          Pg:20
       a) have questionable generalizability to other   kind:c
          cases   Ans:(a)
       b) are subject to reporter bias
       c) are only useful for rare disorders
       d) necessitate breaking confidentiality

11

1.54: The nature-nurture controversy refers to debate over:

a) the relative importance of biological and environmental causes of behavior
b) different parenting styles in different cultures
c) the role of the mother-child bond in psychopathology
d) animalistic urges central to some mental illnesses

MC/Mod
Pg:20
kind:c
Ans:(a)

1.55: The current dominant view on the cause of psychological disorders views abnormal behavior as resulting from:

a) a combination of biological and environmental factors
b) primarily biological factors such as genetics
c) primarily environmental factors such as learning
d) biological factors in less serious cases, environmental factors in more serious cases

MC/Mod
Pg:21
kind:c
Ans:(a)

1.56: A diathesis is a:

a) symptom of mental illness
b) predisposition or vulnerability
c) form of stress
d) biological cause of mental illness

MC/Easy
Pg:21
kind:f
Ans:(b)

1.57: Schizophrenia runs in Katie's family. If Katie has inherited genes associated with schizophrenia, this genetic inheritance represents a:

a) threshold   b) stress
c) diathesis   d) cause

MC/Diff
Pg:21
kind:a
Ans:(c)

1.58: Some psychologists believe that alcoholism results from a genetic predisposition to be addicted to alcohol plus life experiences that drive a person to drink more and more. This type of analysis is an example of:

a) the nature-nurture controversy
b) circular thinking
c) biological etiology
d) the diathesis-stress model

MC/Mod
Pg:21
kind:c
Ans:(d)

12

1.59: Ernest Hemingway suffered from: MC/Easy
Pg:21
kind:f
Ans:(a)

     a) alcoholism   b) bulimia
     c) schizophrenia   d) mania

1.60: The biopsychosocial model of psychopathology: MC/Mod
Pg:21
kind:c
Ans:(b)

     a) is primarily a medical model
     b) holds that biological, psychological, and social influences interact to produce abnormal behavior
     c) says biological causes lead to psychological problems with social outcomes
     d) examines effects of physical illness on psychological health

1.61: Psychopharmacology is: MC/Easy
Pg:24
kind:f
Ans:(b)

     a) research on how various types of medication can cause psychological symptoms as side effects
     b) the use of medication to treat mental illness
     c) a view which holds that substance abuse is a form of mental disorder
     d) a movement among psychologists to earn prescription privileges

1.62: Which of the following is an example of what a cognitive therapist does?   MC/Mod
Pg:24
kind:c
Ans:(c)

     a) uses medication to control thought disorders
     b) studies the neurological basis of thinking and learning
     c) helps patients change illogical thinking and assumptions
     d) works to uncover the unconscious symbolism of unwanted thoughts

1.63: In the Epidemiologic Catchment Area (ECA) study, one out of every five Americans showed active symptoms of at least one mental disorder. Of these people, what proportion had received treatment for the condition in the last few months?   MC/Diff
Pg:24
kind:f
Ans:(b)

     a) 5%   b) 20%
     c) 80%   d) 95%

1.64: Freud's use of hypnosis and free association to treat patients with physical and emotional complaints is an example of:

MC/Diff
Pg:25
kind:c
Ans:(d)

  a) how psychopathology can be psychosomatic
  b) how psychological problems can have biological causes
  c) how useful theories can spawn new therapies
  d) how useful therapies can spawn new theories

1.65: Which is true about the first antipsychotic drugs in the 1950s?

MC/Diff
Pg:25
kind:c
Ans:(c)

  a) they were developed based on theories of the neurochemistry of psychosis
  b) they led to the diathesis-stress model of etiology
  c) their discovery led to speculation about the neurochemistry of psychosis
  d) they had poor success because of biological reductionism

1.66: The first antipsychotic medications in the 1950s were:

MC/Mod
Pg:25
kind:f
Ans:(d)

  a) being used as recreational drugs
  b) neurotransmitters synthesized in the laboratory
  c) neurotransmitters taken from animals
  d) discovered by accident

1.67: Biological reductionism assumes that:

MC/Mod
Pg:25
kind:c
Ans:(b)

  a) mental illness leads to a lowered chance for reproduction
  b) most psychological disorders have an underlying biological problem associated with them
  c) mental illness is caused by reductions in neurotransmitters
  d) biology should be given less attention in clinical psychology

1.68: The idea that every psychological disorder has a   MC/Mod
       more elemental underlying biological cause is an   Pg:25
       idea associated with: kind:c
                                                               Ans:(c)

       a) the diathesis-stress model
       b) the nature-nurture controversy
       c) biological reductionism
       d) the threshold model

True-False Questions

1.69: Unlike psychiatrists, clinical psychologists have a   TF/Easy
       medical degree.   Pg:3
                                                              kind:f
                                                              Ans:False

1.70: Clinical psychologists can treat patients without   TF/Mod
       the supervision of psychiatrists.   Pg:4
                                                              kind:f
                                                              Ans:True

1.71: One example of an hallucination is hearing voices   TF/Mod
       when no other people are present.   Pg:4
                                                              kind:a
                                                              Ans:True

1.72: The distinguishing characteristic of formal thought   TF/Mod
       disorder, or disorganized speech, is not the   Pg:4
       content of what the person is saying but that it is   kind:c
       said in a vague way that is difficult to   Ans:True
       understand.

1.73: Mental disorders are defined in terms of persistent   TF/Mod
       maladaptive behaviors.   Pg:8
                                                              kind:c
                                                              Ans:True

1.74: According to DSM-IV, voluntary artistic and   TF/Diff
       political activities could be considered to be   Pg:9
       manifestations of mental disorder if they result in   kind:c
       social impairment (e.g., imprisonment).   Ans:False

1.75: Eating disorders can be fatal if they are not properly treated, because of their effect on vital organs.

TF/Mod
Pg:13
kind:f
Ans:True

1.76: A dimensional system of classification sees abnormal behavior as fundamentally or qualitatively different from normal behavior.

TF/Mod
Pg:13
kind:c
Ans:False

1.77: The DSM-IV is based on a dimensional, not categorical, approach to classification.

TF/Mod
Pg:14
kind:c
Ans:False

1.78: Incidence is defined as the number of new cases that develop in a population during a specified period of time.

TF/Mod
Pg:14
kind:f
Ans:True

1.79: Prevalence is defined as the number of new cases developing in a population during a specific period of time.

TF/Mod
Pg:14
kind:f
Ans:False

1.80: The symptoms of pellagra have sometimes been mistaken for schizophrenia.

TF/Mod
Pg:14
kind:f
Ans:True

1.81: Anthropological studies show that in nonwestern cultures, "crazy" behavior is viewed as being quite distinct from behavior that is associated with being a shaman or spiritual leader.

TF/Mod
Pg:15
kind:f
Ans:True

1.82: Rates of schizophrenia are much higher in industrialized countries than in developing countries.

TF/Mod
Pg:15
kind:f
Ans:False

1.83: Schizophrenia is about equally common in women and in men.

TF/Mod
Pg:16
kind:f
Ans:True

1.84: The Epidemiologic Catchment Area (ECA) study of mental disorders in the U.S. found that lifetime rates are higher than one-year prevalence rates.

TF/Diff
Pg:16
kind:f
Ans:True

1.85: Epidemiology refers to the study of causes and origins of disorders.

TF/Mod
Pg:16
kind:f
Ans:False

1.86: Case studies are useful for clinical treatment but are not used for research purposes.

TF/Mod
Pg:19
kind:c
Ans:False

1.87: Diathesis is a form of treatment for stress.

TF/Easy
Pg:21
kind:f
Ans:False

1.88: A diathesis is necessarily a biologically-based predisposition.

TF/Mod
Pg:21
kind:c
Ans:False

1.89: The biopsychosocial model of psychopathology holds that biological causes produce psychological problems with social outcomes.

TF/Mod
Pg:21
kind:c
Ans:False

1.90: The biopsychosocial model of etiology is primarily held by psychiatrists, not psychologists.

TF/Mod
Pg:21
kind:c
Ans:False

1.91: It is not unusual for patients with mental disorders to receive medication while they are also involved in psychotherapy.

TF/Mod
Pg:24
kind:f
Ans:True

1.92: The Epidemiologic Catchment Area (ECA) study found that a minority of people with mental illness actually get treatment.

TF/Mod
Pg:24
kind:f
Ans:True

1.93: Definitions of mental disorders are still being debated.

TF/Easy
Pg:26
kind:c
Ans:True

Essay Questions

1.94: Describe the problems that are associated with attempts to define abnormal behavior in terms of (a) subjective distress; (b) statistical rarity; and (c) biological disadvantage.

Answer: (a) The individual may show low insight into the condition, and the behaviors may bother others but not the individual. (b) The cutoff for statistical rarity might have to be arbitrary, and would be different for different disorders. Statistical rarity doesn't address the issue of whether the behavior is harmful or not harmful. In addition, some mental disorders are actually quite common. (c) Not all mental disorders are associated with a clear disadvantage for reproduction or survival, as might be argued for schizophrenia.

ES Difficult Page: 9 kind: c

1.95: Describe what types of categories of behavior are excluded from categorization as mental illness in the DSM-IV, and give an example of each.

Answer: (1) Expected or culturally sanctioned behaviors, such as behavior which occurs as part of mourning rituals; (2) rare or unusual behaviors not associated with personal distress or impairment of social functioning, such as religious expression; (3) voluntary expressions of conflict between the individual and society, such as political protest or controversial artwork.

ES Difficult Page: 9 kind: c

1.96: What is the difference between a categorical approach and a dimensional approach to classification? Use the example of bulimia nervosa to describe how these two systems would be applied to diagnosis.

Answer: (1) The categorical approach is based on the idea of qualitative differences between what is normal and abnormal; the dimensional approach is based on the idea that there are quantitative differences between what is normal and abnormal. (2) In terms of bulimia, a categorical or qualitative approach assumes that bulimics have some trait, such as an inability to perceive internal cues, which makes them different from non-bulimics; the dimensional or quantitative approach assumes that bulimia is an extreme expression of behaviors and attitudes that are also expressed to varying degrees by persons who do not have eating disorders.

ES Difficult Page: 13 kind: c

1.97: Describe the benefits and drawbacks of the use of case studies in clinical psychology.

Answer: (1) Benefits: rich clinical descriptions, especially important if the disorder is rare; can be used to generate hypotheses; associated details can give clues about the nature of mental illness. (2) Drawbacks: can be viewed from many different perspectives; risky to draw general conclusions from a single case.

ES Moderate Pages: 19-20 kind: c

1.98: Discuss the limitations of the idea that the cause of a condition can be inferred from information regarding the efficacy of various treatment approaches that are used to help people who suffer from the condition.

Answer: (1) The symptoms that are treated may be the effect of the condition, not the cause of it. (2) There may be multiple causes for any disorder. (3) It is faulty logic to say that one has a headache because of lack of aspirin.

ES Moderate Pages: 25-26 kind: c

Chapter 2
Causes of Abnormal Behavior:
From Paradigms to Systems

Multiple Choice Questions

2.1: The etiology of a problem is its: MC/Easy
                                                               Pg:32
    a) cause   b) treatment   kind:f
    c) classification   d) paradigm   Ans:(a)

2.2: A way of looking at scientific problems, and views   MC/Mod
     about acceptable scientific methodology, are part   Pg:32
     of: kind:f
                                                               Ans:(d)
    a) a theory   b) an etiology
    c) a diagnosis   d) a paradigm

2.3: Almost all forms of abnormal behavior are thought   MC/Mod
     to be caused by: Pg:32
                                                               kind:f
    a) a single cause   b) genetics   Ans:(c)
    c) multiple factors d) learning

2.4: Hippocrates (460-367 B.C.) believed that insanity   MC/Mod
     was due to: Pg:35
                                                               kind:f
    a) demons   Ans:(b)
    b) an imbalance in body fluids
    c) infection
    d) guilt

2.5: An important scientific advancement in the   MC/Mod
     understanding of the etiology of psychopathology   Pg:35
     occurred in the 19th century, with the discovery of   kind:f
     the cause of: Ans:(b)

    a) schizophrenia   b) general paresis
    c) Alzheimers disease d) depression

2.6: In the 1800s, a form of mental illness called   MC/Mod
     general paresis was discovered to be caused by   Pg:36
     destruction of parts of the central nervous system   kind:f
     due to: Ans:(c)

     a) brain and spine injury
     b) inherited chromosomal abnormality
     c) infection with syphilis
     d) imbalances in neurotransmitters

2.7: When Freud introduced his ideas on the role of   MC/Mod
     early childhood experiences in the development of   Pg:36
     mental illness, the prevailing paradigm was: kind:c
                                                            Ans:(c)
     a) behavioristic   b) experimental
     c) biological   d) humanistic

2.8: Freud was interested in the use of hypnosis to   MC/Mod
     treat hysteria because such treatment seemed to   Pg:36
     demonstrate: kind:c
                                                            Ans:(a)
     a) different levels of conscious awareness
     b) biological causes of psychological problems
     c) benefits of experimental psychology
     d) distinctions between general paresis and other
        disorders

2.9: Freud built his theory of the development of normal   MC/Mod
     and abnormal behavior based on: Pg:37
                                                            kind:c
     a) case histories and introspection   Ans:(a)
     b) experimental tests
     c) biological research
     d) developmental norms

2.10: In Freudian theory, sexual and aggressive drives   MC/Easy
      are part of the mind called the: Pg:37
                                                            kind:f
      a) conscience   b) ego   Ans:(d)
      c) superego   d) id

2.11: According to Freudian theory, the pleasure
principle refers to the idea that:

    a) the conscience makes people feel guilty
    b) unconscious impulses want immediate
       gratification
    c) the ego must cope realistically with the
       external world
    d) societal rules are attempts to govern id
       impulses

MC/Mod
Pg:37
kind:c
Ans:(b)

2.12: According to Freudian theory, the part of the mind
that is roughly equivalent to the conscience is:

    a) the superego   b) the ego
    c) the id   d) defense mechanisms

MC/Easy
Pg:37
kind:f
Ans:(a)

2.13: According to Freudian theory, the reality principle
is the framework of operation of the:

    a) id   b) ego
    c) superego   d) conscience

MC/Mod
Pg:37
kind:f
Ans:(b)

2.14: According to Freud, defense mechanisms serve to
reduce:

    a) psychosis   b) self-actualization
    c) introspection   d) anxiety

MC/Mod
Pg:37
kind:c
Ans:(d)

2.15: According to Freud, a boy resolves forbidden sexual
desire for his mother by:

    a) becoming attracted to girls
    b) identifying with his father
    c) developing aggressive urges toward his mother
    d) developing an Electra complex

MC/Mod
Pg:38
kind:c
Ans:(b)

2.16: The science of psychology was born in 1879 in the
laboratory of:

    a) Pavlov   b) Wundt
    c) Skinner   d) Freud

MC/Easy
Pg:38
kind:f
Ans:(b)

2.17: Early systematic research on the nature of human consciousness occurred in Wundt's laboratory. Wundt asked subjects to:

MC/Mod
Pg:38
kind:f
Ans:(b)

a) undergo hypnosis
b) report in detail about their inner experiences
c) undergo learning trials with classical conditioning
d) undergo learning trials with operant conditioning

2.18: Pavlov rang a bell every time he fed meat powder to dogs. After repeated trials, the dogs began to salivate when they heard the bell, even if there was no food in sight. According to Pavlov's ideas on classical conditioning, the dogs' salivation in the absence of food is called the:

MC/Mod
Pg:38
kind:c
Ans:(b)

a) conditioned stimulus
b) conditioned response
c) unconditioned stimulus
d) unconditioned response

2.19: According to Pavlov's ideas on classical conditioning, extinction occurs when a conditioned stimulus is no longer presented along with:

MC/Mod
Pg:38
kind:c
Ans:(c)

a) a conditioned response
b) an unconditioned response
c) an unconditioned stimulus
d) operant conditioning

2.20: A primary concept in Skinner's principle of operant conditioning is that:

MC/Mod
Pg:39
kind:c
Ans:(c)

a) a conditioned response leads to extinction
b) a conditioned stimulus is neutral
c) behavior is a function of its consequences
d) negative reinforcement is the same as punishment

2.21: According to Skinner's principle of operant
conditioning, what happens when negative
reinforcement is applied?

    a) behavior is punished
    b) behavior increases
    c) behavior decreases
    d) behavior remains at the same level

MC/Mod
Pg:39
kind:c
Ans:(b)

2.22: Your neighbors are playing loud music late at night
and it annoys you. You ask them to turn down the
music and they do. The next time they play loud
music, you call them even sooner. Skinner would
say this happens because:

    a) your assertiveness is like a punishment
    b) the noise was an unconditioned stimulus
    c) the decreased noise negatively reinforced your
       assertiveness
    d) the decreased noise positively reinforced your
       assertiveness

MC/Diff
Pg:39
kind:a
Ans:(c)

2.23: You leave trash in your friend's car after
borrowing it. Later your friend says she won't
loan you the car anymore. According to Skinner,
the next time you borrow a car from someone, you
are less likely to litter because:

    a) losing car privileges was a form of punishment
    b) losing car privileges was a form of response
       cost
    c) littering was negatively reinforced
    d) littering was positively reinforced

MC/Diff
Pg:39
kind:a
Ans:(b)

2.24: Watson (1878-1958) was best known for:

    a) his theory of classical conditioning
    b) his theory of operant conditioning
    c) a humanistic approach
    d) founding behaviorism

MC/Mod
Pg:39
kind:c
Ans:(d)

2.25: In the well known experiment with Little Albert,   MC/Mod
Watson and Rayner (1920) used classical   Pg:39
conditioning to induce fear of a rat in an   kind:c
11-year-old boy. This type of experiment sheds   Ans:(d)
light on Watson's assumption that abnormal behavior
is:

   a) a result of defense mechanisms
   b) produced through reinforcement
   c) a form of displacement
   d) learned in the same way as are normal behaviors

2.26: You get a paper back from your favorite professor.   MC/Mod
You briefly feel angry at the low grade you   Pg:39
received, but this feeling is upsetting because you kind:a
like the professor so much. You quickly turn your   Ans:(d)
attention to other matters. Later that day you
pick a fight with your roommate because of the
unfair manner in which the week's chores were
divided. This is an example of a defense mechanism
called:

   a) projection   b) rationalization
   c) sublimation   d) displacement

2.27: Humanistic psychologists objected to the   MC/Mod
biological, psychoanalytic, and behavioral theories Pg:39
of abnormal behavior because these other approaches kind:c
assume that: Ans:(b)

   a) there is free will
   b) behavior is predictably determined
   c) human nature is inherently good
   d) behavior is a paradigm

2.28: A paradigm is: MC/Mod
                                                      Pg:40
   a) a set of guidelines about treatment   kind:c
   b) an explicitly positive view of human nature   Ans:(d)
   c) a belief in determinism
   d) a theory and assumptions about how to test it

2.29: The psychoanalytic paradigm is criticized for: MC/Mod
                                                      Pg:40
   a) being devoid of theory   kind:c
   b) failing to offer testable hypotheses   Ans:(b)
   c) overemphasizing the medical model
   d) being a philosophy rather than a theory

25

2.30: Holism, a central principle of systems theory, is the idea that:

    a) the whole is greater than the sum of its parts
    b) behavior is determined
    c) human nature is basically good
    d) humans have free will

MC/Easy
Pg:41
kind:c
Ans:(a)

2.31: The idea that ultimate explanations for abnormal behavior are found when problems are analyzed in terms of their smallest possible components is known as:

    a) reductionism   b) holism
    c) a paradigm   d) determinism

MC/Easy
Pg:42
kind:c
Ans:(a)

2.32: Cybernetics is a systemic process based on:

    a) feedback loops
    b) developmental psychopathology
    c) linear causality
    d) reductionism

MC/Easy
Pg:43
kind:f
Ans:(a)

2.33: Developmental psychopathology is a new approach to abnormal psychology that emphasized the importance of analyzing behavior in terms of:

    a) homeostasis and cybernetics
    b) early childhood trauma
    c) learned patterns that are more ingrained over time
    d) comparing individual behavior to age-based norms

MC/Mod
Pg:44
kind:c
Ans:(d)

2.34: A pattern of behavior that is apparent before a disorder develops is called:

    a) a prognosis
    b) homeostasis
    c) a premorbid pattern
    d) a developmental norm

MC/Mod
Pg:44
kind:f
Ans:(c)

2.35: Two psychologists are discussing a patient with psychosis. One psychologist asks the other what the prognosis is. The psychologist wants to know:

    a) what the diagnosis is
    b) what the premorbid history was
    c) the developmental norm for psychosis
    d) the predicted outcome

MC/Mod
Pg:44
kind:c
Ans:(d)

2.36: A neuron is a:

    a) synapse
    b) brain structure
    c) physiological impairment
    d) brain cell

MC/Easy
Pg:45
kind:f
Ans:(d)

2.37: The cell body of the neuron is called the:

    a) dendrite   b) axon
    c) soma   d) synapse

MC/Easy
Pg:45
kind:f
Ans:(c)

2.38: A synapse is a:

    a) nerve cell
    b) cell body
    c) fluid-filled gap between neurons
    d) chemical substance in the brain

MC/Easy
Pg:45
kind:f
Ans:(c)

2.39: The part of the neuron that receives messages from other cells is the:

    a) soma   b) axon
    c) terminal button d) dendrite

MC/Easy
Pg:45
kind:f
Ans:(d)

2.40: Information is transmitted between nerve cells by means of:

    a) changes in electrical potential along the axon
    b) changes in electrical potential in the synapse
    c) release of neurotransmitters at the synapse
    d) release of neurotransmitters along the axon

MC/Mod
Pg:45
kind:c
Ans:(c)

2.41: Sometimes some neurotransmitters in the synapse return to the terminal buttons of the neuron that released them. This is known as:

    a) neuromodulation
    b) dualism
    c) reuptake
    d) electrical potential

MC/Easy
Pg:45
kind:f
Ans:(c)

2.42: Dualism refers to the idea that:

    a) mind and body are separate
    b) the brain is made up of structures and functions
    c) humans are influenced by free will and determinism
    d) the whole is greater than the sum of its parts

MC/Mod
Pg:46
kind:c
Ans:(a)

2.43: The part of the hindbrain that coordinates body movements is the:

    a) cerebellum
    b) medulla
    c) pons
    d) reticular activating system

MC/Mod
Pg:46
kind:f
Ans:(a)

2.44: The basic bodily functions such as heart rate, stages of sleep, and balance are regulated by the:

    a) forebrain   b) midbrain
    c) hindbrain   d) corpus callosum

MC/Easy
Pg:46
kind:f
Ans:(c)

2.45: Motor activities associated with fighting and sexual behavior are controlled by the:

    a) midbrain   b) forebrain
    c) hindbrain   d) corpus callosum

MC/Easy
Pg:47
kind:f
Ans:(a)

2.46: The reticular activating system regulates:

    a) sex drive   b) aggression
    c) sleeping and waking d) cognitive processes

MC/Easy
Pg:47
kind:f
Ans:(c)

2.47: Regulation of emotion is a central role of the: MC/Easy
Pg:47

    a) limbic system
    b) reticular activating system
    c) cerebellum
    d) corpus callosum

kind:f
Ans:(a)

2.48: The thalamus and hypothalamus are part of the: MC/Easy
Pg:47

    a) limbic system
    b) reticular activating system
    c) cerebellum
    d) corpus callosum

kind:f
Ans:(a)

2.49: Communication and coordination between the 2 MC/Easy
hemispheres takes place at the: Pg:47

kind:f

    a) cerebellum   b) corpus callosum Ans:(b)
    c) limbic system   d) spine

2.50: The 4 ventricles in the brain are: MC/Easy
Pg:47

    a) large nerve cells connecting parts of the brain kind:f
    b) the forebrain, midbrain, hindbrain, and Ans:(d)
       cerebellum
    c) veins carrying blood to the brain
    d) chambers filled with cerebrospinal fluid

2.51: The most sophisticated human abilities of memory MC/Easy
and the integration of sensory and motor functions Pg:47
are the responsibility of the: kind:f

Ans:(d)

    a) corpus callosum   b) cerebellum
    c) ventricles   d) cerebral cortex

2.52: The endocrine system is a collection of: MC/Easy
Pg:48

    a) glands   b) neurons kind:f
    c) brain structures   d) ventricles Ans:(a)

2.53: The central nervous system includes:

    a) the somatic and autonomic nervous systems
    b) the sympathetic and parasympathetic nervous
       systems
    c) the pituitary, thyroid, and adrenal glands
    d) the brain and spinal cord

MC/Easy
Pg:48
kind:f
Ans:(d)

2.54: You move your arm to scratch your leg. This
     behavior is regulated by which part of the nervous
     system?

    a) sympathetic   b) parasympathetic
    c) autonomic   d) somatic

MC/Mod
Pg:48
kind:a
Ans:(d)

2.55: In the autonomic nervous system, increased arousal
     is associated with activation of the:

    a) somatic nervous system
    b) central nervous system
    c) sympathetic nervous system
    d) parasympathetic nervous system

MC/Mod
Pg:49
kind:f
Ans:(c)

2.56: Optimal nervous system energy is described by:

    a) homeostasis in sympathetic and parasympathetic
       nervous systems
    b) somatic nervous system controlling autonomic
       nervous system
    c) equal involvement of the central and peripheral
       nervous systems
    d) balance in the activity of neurotransmitters
       and neuromodulators

MC/Mod
Pg:49
kind:c
Ans:(a)

2.57: Behavior geneticists study:

    a) specific genes and their hereditary functions
    b) biochemical chromosomal abnormalities
    c) genotypes
    d) global genetic influences on human behavior

MC/Mod
Pg:49
kind:f
Ans:(d)

2.58: A phenotype is:

    a) a genetic structure
    b) a pattern of dominant and recessive genes
    c) a description of chromosomal abnormality
    d) a set of observable traits

MC/Easy
Pg:50
kind:f
Ans:(d)

2.59: As more genes are involved in determining a trait, the trait is likely to be one that is:

MC/Diff
Pg:50
kind:c
Ans:(d)

a) phenotypical
b) abnormal or pathological
c) easily classified as either present or absent
d) continuously distributed

2.60: If a trait is entirely genetically determined, which of the following could be expected in a twin study of monozygotic (MZ) and dizygotic (DZ) twins?

MC/Mod
Pg:51
kind:c
Ans:(c)

a) DZ twins would have 0% concordance
b) DZ twins would have the same concordance as MZ twins
c) MZ twins would have 100% concordance
d) MZ twins would have 50% concordance

2.61: In a study of twins, a researcher finds that 40% of dizygotic (DZ) twins and 40% of monozygotic (MZ) twins share a trait. The researcher should conclude that the trait appears to be:

MC/Diff
Pg:51
kind:a
Ans:(b)

a) genetically determined
b) environmentally determined
c) normally distributed
d) 60% concordant

2.62: If both monozygotic (MZ) and dizygotic (DZ) twins show a high concordance rate for a disorder, it can be concluded that the disorder is caused by:

MC/Diff
Pg:51
kind:c
Ans:(b)

a) genetics
b) shared environmental experiences
c) recessive genes
d) chromosomal abnormalities

2.63: A twin pair is concordant when:

MC/Mod
Pg:51
kind:c
Ans:(a)

a) both twins have the same disorder
b) both twins were raised similarly
c) one twin has a disorder and the other twin does not
d) the twins share 100% of their genetic material

2.64: In family incidence studies, the proband is:

    a) the rate of concordance among family members
    b) the disorder being studied
    c) a set of characteristic symptoms in the family
    d) one member of the family who is identified as
       normal or ill

MC/Mod
Pg:52
kind:c
Ans:(d)

2.65: According to Maslow's theory of a hierarchy of human needs, the most fundamental human need is:

    a) love   b) esteem
    c) physical survival   d) self-actualization

MC/Mod
Pg:53
kind:f
Ans:(c)

2.66: According to Maslow, self-actualization is:

    a) a learned selfishness necessary to survive
    b) an innate need to fulfill one's potential
    c) a preoccupation with meeting basic biological
       needs
    d) a stage when one does not need love or
       belongingness

MC/Mod
Pg:54
kind:c
Ans:(b)

2.67: Bowlby believed that attachments form because they:

    a) are reinforcing
    b) have survival value
    c) fulfill drives for sex and aggression
    d) are part of self-actualization

MC/Mod
Pg:54
kind:c
Ans:(b)

2.68: The selective relationship that develops between the mother and offspring in the first hours of life among some species such as birds is called:

    a) attachment   b) affiliation
    c) proximity   d) imprinting

MC/Easy
Pg:54
kind:f
Ans:(d)

2.69: One baby is placid and smiley; the other is active and disagreeable. This difference in style is a difference of:

    a) temperament   b) attachment
    c) affiliation   d) motivation

MC/Mod
Pg:55
kind:c
Ans:(a)

2.70: According to Ainsworth and Bowlby, anxious attachments develop during the first year of life because of:

    a) temperament differences
    b) modeling
    c) low self-actualization
    d) inconsistent parenting

MC/Mod
Pg:56
kind:c
Ans:(d)

2.71: According to research, children show the best adjustment when their parents are:

    a) self-actualized
    b) of similar temperament
    c) agreeable and open to experience
    d) firm and loving

MC/Mod
Pg:56
kind:c
Ans:(d)

2.72: Children can learn abnormal or normal behavior through modeling. Modeling is learning based on:

    a) imitation
    b) operant conditioning
    c) classical conditioning
    d) social cognition

MC/Easy
Pg:56
kind:f
Ans:(a)

2.73: Some forms of psychopathology are associated with errors in attribution. This type of error has to do with:

    a) perceived causes
    b) the identification process
    c) modeling
    d) attachment

MC/Easy
Pg:57
kind:f
Ans:(a)

2.74: According to Freud, identification is a process by which children:

    a) recognize some adults as parents
    b) imitate adults' behavior and adopt their values
    c) develop an ego
    d) become aware of their own sexuality

MC/Mod
Pg:57
kind:f
Ans:(b)

2.75: Self-schema are: MC/Mod
                                                           Pg:58
   a) early forms of identification   kind:c
   b) cognitions about the self   Ans:(b)
   c) patterns of relating to others
   d) ego defenses

2.76: According to Albert Ellis, an advocate of rational MC/Mod
      emotive therapy, psychological distress is caused   Pg:58
      by: kind:c
                                                           Ans:(a)
   a) irrational beliefs about the self
   b) poorly integrated identity
   c) lack of internalized standards of conduct
   d) lack of self-actualization

2.77: Socialization is a process whereby children develop: MC/Easy
                                                           Pg:58
   a) identity   b) self-control   kind:f
   c) self-schema   d) self-concept   Ans:(b)

2.78: Albert Bandura emphasized the importance of   MC/Easy
      self-efficacy for psychological wellbeing.   Pg:58
      Self-efficacy is a sense of the self as: kind:f
                                                           Ans:(a)
   a) able to achieve goals
   b) an integrated whole
   c) worthy of love
   d) rational

2.79: One important characteristic of Erikson's theory of MC/Mod
      psychosocial development is the idea that: Pg:59
                                                           kind:c
   a) children ages 5-12 are in a period of latency   Ans:(c)
   b) there are no stages in development
   c) development does not end in adolescence
   d) developmental changes are quantitative, not
      qualitative

2.80: A 10-year-old child normally copes effectively at   MC/Easy
      school. One day under stress, he curls up on the   Pg:59
      floor and begins to suck his thumb. This is an   kind:a
      example of: Ans:(b)

   a) fixation   b) regression
   c) latency   d) transition

2.81: According to labeling theory, emotional disorders and abnormal behavior are created by:

    a) societal expectations
    b) irrational self-schema
    c) fixation and regression
    d) developmental transitions

MC/Mod
Pg:60
kind:c
Ans:(a)

2.82: A child overhears her teacher call her a "troublemaker." The child then stops trying to please the teacher, and actually gets in more trouble. This is known as:

    a) fixation
    b) regression
    c) a developmental transition
    d) a self-fulfilling prophesy

MC/Mod
Pg:60
kind:a
Ans:(d)

2.83: Correlation coefficients always range between:

    a) -1 and +1   b) 0 and 1
    c) 0 and 100   d) -100 and +100

MC/Easy
Pg:61
kind:f
Ans:(a)

2.84: Which of the following correlation coefficients shows the strongest association between 2 variables?

    a) -0.8   b) -0.1
    c) +0.2   d) +0.7

MC/Easy
Pg:61
kind:f
Ans:(a)

True-False Questions

2.85: Abnormal behavior has multifactorial causes.

TF/Easy
Pg:32
kind:f
Ans:True

2.86: According to Freudian theory, the job of the ego is to mediate between the id and the superego.

TF/Easy
Pg:37
kind:f
Ans:True

2.87: The name most closely associated with classical conditioning is Skinner.

TF/Easy
Pg:38
kind:f
Ans:False

2.88: Negative reinforcement is the same as punishment.

TF/Easy
Pg:39
kind:c
Ans:False

2.89: An important characteristic of humanistic psychology is a belief in determinism.

TF/Easy
Pg:39
kind:f
Ans:False

2.90: A basic idea of systems theory is that causality is linear.

TF/Easy
Pg:43
kind:f
Ans:False

2.91: Psychosocial development continues throughout adult life.

TF/Easy
Pg:44
kind:f
Ans:True

2.92: Anatomy is concerned with biological structures, and physiology is concerned with biological functions.

TF/Easy
Pg:45
kind:f
Ans:True

2.93: Information transmitted within a neuron is due to changes in chemical substances at the synapse.

TF/Easy
Pg:45
kind:f
Ans:False

2.94: Neuromodulators are chemicals that influence communication among many neurons.

TF/Mod
Pg:46
kind:f
Ans:True

2.95: The largest part of the human brain is the forebrain.

TF/Easy
Pg:47
kind:f
Ans:True

2.96: In general the left hemisphere is involved in language and related functions.

TF/Easy
Pg:47
kind:f
Ans:True

2.97: The endocrine system produces psychophysiological changes by releasing hormones into the blood stream.

TF/Easy
Pg:48
kind:f
Ans:True

2.98: Chromosomes are located on genes.

TF/Easy
Pg:49
kind:f
Ans:False

2.99: Humans normally have 23 pairs of chromosomes.

TF/Easy
Pg:49
kind:f
Ans:True

2.100: Like all siblings, dizygotic (DZ) twins share 50% of their genes on average.

TF/Mod
Pg:51
kind:f
Ans:True

2.101: If a trait is genetically caused, the environment can have no impact on its expression.

TF/Mod
Pg:52
kind:f
Ans:False

2.102: Abraham Maslow is known for founding behavioral psychology.

TF/Easy
Pg:53
kind:f
Ans:False

2.103: A correlation of +1.0 or -1.0 indicates causality.

TF/Easy
Pg:61
kind:f
Ans:False

2.104: Cultural relativity is the idea that the definition of abnormal behavior is the same in any culture.

TF/Easy
Pg:66
kind:f
Ans:False

Essay Questions

2.105: Describe how a paradigm can both direct and misdirect scientists.

Answer: A paradigm can suggest ways to look for answers to questions and the methodology to test ideas. On the other hand, a paradigm works under assumptions that may be appropriate for one theory but that may hinder the discovery of solutions to other problems, because of a limiting mindset.

ES Moderate Page: 40 kind: c

2.106: Define reductionism. Discuss the limitations of the reductionistic idea that if a depletion of certain chemicals in the brain accompanies depression, then the depletion must be the cause of the depression.

Answer: Reductionism is the belief that ultimate causes rest in the smallest units of analysis. However, in the case of depression, just because chemicals are a small unit of analysis does not mean that they are a more likely causal element. Broader elements such as behavior, relationships, and negative cognitions associated with depression could also cause chemical changes in the brain.

ES Moderate Page: 42 kind: c

2.107: Define homeostasis and describe how it applies to psychological, not just biological, processes.

Answer: Homeostasis is the tendency to maintain a steady state. It is related to the idea of cybernetics, that input influences subsequent adjustments in a process of feedback. An example in psychological terms is that an individual seeks a moderate, optimal level of stimulation; e.g., a person deprived of sensory input may begin to hallucinate, or a person who is overstimulated may withdraw.

ES Moderate Page: 44 kind: c

2.108: Discuss the implications of the idea that most forms of psychopathology are polygenic.

Answer: Polygenic traits are continuously distributed, and thus polygenic abnormal traits are on a continuum with normal traits. This may make it difficult to determine the threshold of abnormality, which may be a question of degree rather than qualitative differences. This can make diagnosis less reliable, and complicates research on etiology.

ES   Moderate   Page: 50   kind: c

2.109: The assumption that the environment affects dizygotic (DZ) twins in the same way it influences monozygotic (MZ) twins has been criticized. Describe this criticism and the research methodology used to address it.

Answer: The criticism is that there may be greater concordance among MZ twins in part because they are treated more similarly than are DZ twins. To address this, adoption studies have been conducted. If the concordance is higher for biological relatives than for adoptive relatives, this points to genetic involvement in the trait.

ES   Moderate   Page: 52   kind: c

2.110: What have researchers identified as the 5 basic bipolar dimensions of personality?

Answer: (1) extraversion (active and talkative vs. passive and reserved)
(2) agreeable (trusting and kind vs. hostile and selfish)
(3) conscientiousness (organized and reliable vs. careless and neglectful)
(4) neuroticism (nervous and moody vs. calm and pleasant)
(5) openness to experience (imaginative and curious vs. shallow and imperceptive)

ES   Moderate   Page: 56   kind: c

2.111: Depression has been linked with errors or distortions in information processing. Describe some of these errors.

Answer: Learned helplessness occurs when an individual wrongly attributes bad events to internal, global, and stable causes. Cognitive errors also occur because of inaccurate, negative generalizations about the self.

ES   Moderate   Page: 57   kind: c

2.112: It would be a mistake to interpret a high correlation between
        anxiety and low self-esteem as meaning that low-self esteem causes
        anxiety. Discuss the alternative interpretations.

Answer: Reverse causality: anxiety could cause low self-esteem.
        Third variable: some other variable such as depression could
        cause both anxiety and low self-esteem.

        ES Moderate Page: 61 kind: c

2.113: Discuss how gender roles affect the development, expression, and
        consequences of psychopathology.

Answer: Gender roles may CAUSE problems; e.g. women are raised to show
        dependency and helplessness, which may cause depression. Gender
        roles may affect the EXPRESSION of problems; e.g. it is socially
        acceptable for women to show depression, and for men to show
        physical illness. Gender roles can affect the CONSEQUENCES of
        problems; e.g. once a phobia develops, it is socially acceptable
        for women, but not men, to continue to avoid the feared object,
        and this may exacerbate the problem for women.

        ES Moderate Page: 65 kind: c

Chapter 3
Treatment of Psychological Disorders

Multiple Choice Questions

3.1: Psychotherapy outcome research on psychodynamic, behavioral, and humanistic approaches shows that:

    a) the psychodynamic approach is far more effective
    b) the behavioral approach is far more effective
    c) the humanistic approach is far more effective
    d) each is more beneficial than no treatment

MC/Mod
Pg:73
kind:c
Ans:(d)

3.2: Psychotherapy process research suggests that the outcome of therapy may depend less on the therapist's theoretical orientation than on:

    a) the effectiveness of medication
    b) the type of presenting problem
    c) the patient's defense mechanisms
    d) the special relationship between therapist and client

MC/Mod
Pg:73
kind:c
Ans:(d)

3.3: Eclectic therapists:

    a) adhere strongly to one paradigm of therapy
    b) are biologically oriented
    c) tailor their approach to the client or the disorder
    d) are paraprofessionals

MC/Easy
Pg:73
kind:f
Ans:(c)

3.4: The goal of psychodynamic therapy is most typically described as:

    a) changing psychological experience with the use of medication
    b) applying psychological research to foster learning of new behaviors
    c) promoting awareness of what was unconscious
    d) encouraging acceptance of individual responsibility

MC/Easy
Pg:73
kind:c
Ans:(c)

3.5: The type of therapy most associated with an emphasis on free will and individual responsibility is:

    a) humanistic   b) behavioral
    c) biological   d) psychodynamic

MC/Mod
Pg:74
kind:f
Ans:(a)

3.6: A therapist tells a patient that she is thinking and acting like a depressed person, and thus it is not surprising that she feels depressed. The therapist is most likely to be working within which theoretical framework?

    a) psychodynamic   b) behavioral
    c) biological   d) humanistic

MC/Mod
Pg:76
kind:a
Ans:(b)

3.7: A therapist tells a patient that he is not being genuine and not being himself. The therapist encourages the patient to make life choices based on his true feelings. Within which theoretical framework is the therapist most likely working?

    a) psychodynamic   b) behavioral
    c) humanistic   d) biological

MC/Mod
Pg:76
kind:a
Ans:(c)

3.8: An ancient practice called trephining sought to treat mental illness by:

    a) chipping a hole in the skull to let spirits escape
    b) dunking suspected witches in water
    c) confining patients in "insane asylums"
    d) performing sacrifices

MC/Easy
Pg:77
kind:f
Ans:(a)

3.9: Hippocrates, who lived around 400 B.C., recommended what treatment for mental illness?

    a) rest, exercise, healthy diet
    b) trephining
    c) dunking in water
    d) spiritual exorcism

MC/Easy
Pg:77
kind:f
Ans:(a)

3.10: The scientific beginnings of the biological treatment of mental disorders can be traced to the discovery of the diagnosis and cure for general paresis. In which century did this occur?

    a) 17th   b) 18th
    c) 19th   d) 20th

MC/Easy
Pg:77
kind:f
Ans:(c)

3.11: The experiment is the most powerful scientific method because it:

    a) is correlational in nature
    b) can establish cause and effect
    c) is conducted in a laboratory
    d) is statistically significant

MC/Easy
Pg:78
kind:c
Ans:(b)

3.12: In an experiment, a researcher gives some patients therapy, gives others medication, and puts others on a waiting list. The researcher then measures how depressed the patients are feeling after 6 months. The independent variable in this scenario is:

    a) improvement in depression
    b) time span of 6 months
    c) kind of treatment received
    d) the number of patients

MC/Mod
Pg:78
kind:a
Ans:(c)

3.13: The outcomes or changes produced by manipulation of an experimental variable are known as:

    a) the hypothesis
    b) random assignment
    c) the independent variable
    d) the dependent variable

MC/Mod
Pg:78
kind:c
Ans:(d)

3.14: Conventionally, a research finding is considered to be statistically significant if:

    a) there has been substantial change in the independent variable
    b) the hypothesis was supported
    c) such a result would only occur 5% of the time by chance
    d) the subjects were randomly assigned

MC/Mod
Pg:78
kind:c
Ans:(c)

3.15: In the 19th century, general paresis was discovered   MC/Easy
      to be caused by: Pg:79
                                                               kind:f
      a) head injury   b) syphilis   Ans:(b)
      c) recessive genes   d) trephining

3.16: A study of the effectiveness of different forms of   MC/Diff
      psychotherapy could be said to have high internal   Pg:79
      validity if: kind:c
                                                               Ans:(a)
      a) patient improvement can be attributed to the
         psychotherapy, and not to other factors
      b) the findings can be generalized to other types
         of patients
      c) the results are statistically significant
      d) the independent variable is confounded with
         other factors

3.17: If the results of a study are easily generalizable   MC/Diff
      to other circumstances, the study is said to: Pg:79
                                                               kind:c
      a) be confounded   Ans:(d)
      b) be statistically significant
      c) have high internal validity
      d) have high external validity

3.18: Electroconvulsive therapy (ECT) was originally used   MC/Mod
      based on the erroneous assumption that: Pg:80
                                                               kind:f
      a) resulting memory loss would cure schizophrenia   Ans:(d)
      b) schizophrenia was caused by the brain only
         using 1 hemisphere
      c) schizophrenia prevented epileptic seizures
      d) epileptic seizures prevented schizophrenia

3.19: The psychosurgical technique of prefrontal lobotomy   MC/Mod
      was discredited because of frequent and severe side   Pg:80
      effects, including: kind:f
                                                               Ans:(c)
      a) induced epilepsy
      b) anxiety
      c) loss of emotional responsiveness
      d) mania

44

3.20: Some psychologists believe it is unethical to accept sexual offenders for treatment because:

    a) treatment would be coercive
    b) there is little research evidence that treatment would work
    c) sexual offenders should be jailed
    d) treatment would involve deception

MC/Mod
Pg:81
kind:c
Ans:(b)

3.21: Antipsychotic medications help eliminate delusions and hallucinations among people suffering from schizophrenia. When antipsychotic medications are given to non-schizophrenic people, they:

    a) cause disorientation
    b) are addictive
    c) cause delusions and hallucinations
    d) have no effect

MC/Mod
Pg:82
kind:f
Ans:(a)

3.22: Prozac, a medication that has outsold all other prescription medications in the 1990s, is:

    a) an antianxiety medication
    b) an antipsychotic medication
    c) an antidepressant medication
    d) a tranquilizer

MC/Easy
Pg:82
kind:f
Ans:(c)

3.23: Breuer's "cathartic method" provided relief for psychological symptoms through helping patients to express their feelings while:

    a) using free association
    b) under the influence of "truth serum"
    c) under hypnosis
    d) using systematic desensitization

MC/Mod
Pg:84
kind:c
Ans:(c)

3.24: Free association refers to:

    a) talking freely about whatever comes to mind
    b) a defense mechanism seen in personality disorders
    c) less confined settings in modern psychiatric hospitals
    d) the effectiveness of psychoactive medications

MC/Easy
Pg:84
kind:c
Ans:(a)

3.25: Freud believed the true benefit of discussing forbidden topics to be:

    a) emotional catharsis
    b) discovery of childhood trauma
    c) that it could induce hypnosis
    d) that clues were revealed about the unconscious mind

MC/Mod
Pg:84
kind:c
Ans:(d)

3.26: In psychoanalysis, interpretation is something that:

    a) guides the therapist's thinking, but isn't shared with the patient
    b) the patient shares with the therapist to explain her own behavior
    c) the therapist shares with the patient to help her understand her own behavior
    d) is used to induce catharsis

MC/Mod
Pg:84
kind:c
Ans:(c)

3.27: Therapeutic neutrality is viewed as essential in:

    a) Freudian psychoanalysis
    b) rational emotive therapy
    c) client-centered therapy
    d) in vivo desensitization

MC/Mod
Pg:84
kind:c
Ans:(a)

3.28: Which of the following best exemplifies the psychanalytic idea of transference?

    a) a patient begins to use healthier defenses
    b) a therapist's interpretation increases a patient's insight
    c) catharsis brings emotional healing
    d) a patient who is angry at his mother becomes angry at the therapist

MC/Mod
Pg:85
kind:c
Ans:(d)

3.29: One difference between psychanalytic and psychodynamic therapists is that in psychodynamic therapy:

    a) treatment usually lasts longer
    b) the therapist if often more engaged and directive
    c) there is a greater emphasis on the id
    d) there is more focus on original Freudian theory

MC/Mod
Pg:85
kind:c
Ans:(b)

3.30: Erikson's theory of psychosocial stages of
development held that:

    a) the individual's personality changes due to
       social conflicts
    b) personality patterns are fixed during the first
       few years of life
    c) humans have an inborn need for attachment
    d) development means the eradication of defense
       mechanisms

MC/Mod
Pg:86
kind:c
Ans:(a)

3.31: Bowlby's contribution to contemporary thought about
the interpersonal influences on personality and
psychopathology was the idea that humans form
attachments because:

    a) attachments decrease primary drives such as
       hunger and thirst
    b) dependency fosters defense mechanisms
    c) humans have an inborn need to form close
       relationships
    d) humans have an unconscious drive to reproduce

MC/Mod
Pg:86
kind:c
Ans:(c)

3.32: A key figure in developing behaviorism in the U.S.
was:

    a) John Bowlby
    b) John Watson
    c) Karen Horney
    d) Harry Stack Sullivan

MC/Easy
Pg:87
kind:f
Ans:(b)

3.33: The key idea in behavior therapy is that:

    a) old psychological defenses can be replaced with
       new defenses
    b) abnormal behavior is caused by difficult early
       relationships
    c) abnormal behavior is learned and can be
       unlearned
    d) individuals are free to determine their own
       lives

MC/Mod
Pg:87
kind:c
Ans:(c)

3.34: A type of therapy that emphasizes empirical   MC/Mod
      evaluation and the application of psychological   Pg:87
      science to treating clinical problems is: kind:c
                                                          Ans:(d)
      a) psychoanalytic therapy
      b) ego analysis
      c) humanistic therapy
      d) behavior therapy

3.35: Systematic desensitization is a therapy technique   MC/Mod
      based on: Pg:88
                                                          kind:f
      a) operant conditioning   Ans:(b)
      b) classical conditioning
      c) cognitive behavior therapy
      d) ego analysis

3.36: The learning process in systematic desensitization MC/Mod
      is the pairing of: Pg:88
                                                          kind:c
      a) flooding with in vivo experience   Ans:(d)
      b) unpleasant response with addictive stimuli
      c) contingency management with token economy
      d) feared stimulus with relaxation response

3.37: In vivo desensitization involves being gradually   MC/Mod
      exposed to a feared object while: Pg:88
                                                          kind:c
      a) relaxed in a laboratory setting   Ans:(b)
      b) relaxed in a natural or real-life setting
      c) experiencing intense anxiety in a laboratory
         setting
      d) experiencing intense anxiety in a natural or
         real-life setting

3.38: The key to the technique of flooding in the   MC/Mod
      treatment of phobia is: Pg:88
                                                          kind:c
      a) relaxation throughout exposure   Ans:(d)
      b) gradual exposure
      c) contingency management
      d) preventing avoidance

48

3.39: A treatment commonly used to help smokers stop smoking is:

    a) systematic desensitization
    b) aversion therapy
    c) in vivo desensitization
    d) contingency management

MC/Easy
Pg:88
kind:f
Ans:(b)

3.40: A token economy system in a psychiatric hospital is used to:

    a) reduce reliance on outside income
    b) foster dependency among patients
    c) increase supply and demand of therapy activities
    d) reinforce appropriate behavior

MC/Easy
Pg:89
kind:c
Ans:(d)

3.41: Cognitive behavior therapy is known for its focus on:

    a) studying only observable behaviors, not thoughts about behaviors
    b) the importance of unobservable thought processes on behavior
    c) assertiveness training
    d) systematic desensitization

MC/Easy
Pg:90
kind:f
Ans:(b)

3.42: An attribution is:

    a) an example of a defense mechanism
    b) the perceived cause of something
    c) a personality trait
    d) a change made over the course of therapy

MC/Easy
Pg:90
kind:f
Ans:(b)

3.43: A cognitive behavioral therapist attempts to change a patient's attributions. Which of the following is an example of what the therapist would be most likely to try to get the patient to do?

    a) stop blaming herself for bad things
    b) use rationalization rather than denial
    c) form a secure attachment with the therapist
    d) relax when near a feared object

MC/Mod
Pg:90
kind:a
Ans:(a)

3.44: The point of self-instruction training is to help:

    a) children learn to internalize rules of appropriate behavior
    b) adults to be more assertive
    c) depressed persons to change their attributions
    d) patients to engage in collaborative empiricism

MC/Mod
Pg:91
kind:c
Ans:(a)

3.45: Beck's cognitive therapy was developed specifically as a treatment for:

    a) anxiety   b) depression
    c) impulsivity   d) low assertiveness

MC/Easy
Pg:91
kind:f
Ans:(b)

3.46: A difference between rational emotive therapy (RET) and Beck's cognitive therapy is that in RET:

    a) the therapist directly challenges irrational beliefs
    b) usually only depression is treated
    c) the therapist helps the patient recognize irrationality without direct confrontation
    d) operant conditioning is used

MC/Mod
Pg:91
kind:c
Ans:(a)

3.47: A major difference between a psychodynamic approach and a behavioral approach is that:

    a) behavior therapy focuses on treatment regardless of causes
    b) the course of behavior therapy depends on theoretical assumptions about the nature of psychopathology
    c) psychodynamic approaches have been better researched
    d) psychodynamic therapy focuses on direct education of the patient

MC/Mod
Pg:91
kind:c
Ans:(a)

3.48: Humanistic therapists believe that emotional distress results from:

    a) insecure attachment
    b) learned abnormal behaviors
    c) ineffective defense mechanisms
    d) frustration and alienation

MC/Mod
Pg:92
kind:c
Ans:(d)

3.49: Client-centered therapy is associated with the concepts of:

    a) operant conditioning and classical conditioning
    b) transference and countertransference
    c) empathy and unconditional positive regard
    d) insight and interpretation

MC/Mod
Pg:92
kind:c
Ans:(c)

3.50: A gestalt therapist is likely to:

    a) confront a client's phoniness to provoke emotion
    b) provide unconditional positive regard
    c) maintain therapeutic neutrality
    d) interpret transference

MC/Mod
Pg:93
kind:c
Ans:(a)

3.51: Existential therapy emphasizes:

    a) unconditional positive regard
    b) ego analysis
    c) therapeutic neutrality
    d) finding meaning in life

MC/Easy
Pg:93
kind:f
Ans:(d)

3.52: Meta-analysis is a:

    a) form of psychoanalysis
    b) case study
    c) way of measuring increases and decreases in behavior
    d) statistical technique for combining the results of many studies

MC/Easy
Pg:94
kind:f
Ans:(d)

3.53: Meta-analytic studies combining the results of many studies of outcomes after therapy show an effect size of 0.85. This means:

    a) 85% of patients improve in therapy
    b) therapy does not work for 15% of patients
    c) therapy is almost 100% better than no therapy
    d) patients function .85 of a standard deviation better than controls

MC/Mod
Pg:94
kind:f
Ans:(d)

3.54: Spontaneous remission refers to a patient:

    a) getting worse without therapy
    b) getting worse with therapy
    c) getting better without therapy
    d) getting better with therapy

MC/Easy
Pg:94
kind:f
Ans:(c)

3.55: Research indicates that improvement in therapy is most likely to occur:

    a) among intelligent, successful people, after several years
    b) among intelligent, successful people, in the first few months
    c) among the most disturbed clients, after several years
    d) among the most disturbed clients, in the first few months

MC/Mod
Pg:95
kind:c
Ans:(b)

3.56: Compared to humanistic and psychodynamic therapies, behavior therapy may be particularly effective in the treatment of:

    a) anxiety disorders
    b) depression
    c) schizophrenia
    d) personality disorders

MC/Easy
Pg:96
kind:f
Ans:(a)

3.57: Research comparing behavioral and psychoanalytic therapies has found that:

    a) therapist empathy only matters in psychoanalytic therapy
    b) behavior therapists offer fewer interpretations
    c) psychodynamic therapy is more effective with severe cases
    d) clients see the therapist-client relationship as most important to outcome, in both types of therapy

MC/Easy
Pg:97
kind:c
Ans:(d)

3.58: Psychotherapy process researchers study:

    a) which theoretical perspective on therapy is most effective
    b) patients' psychophysiological reactions during therapy
    c) how therapy is managed by the health care system
    d) qualities of the therapist-client relationship that predict success

3.59: Analysis of the commonalities across different forms of therapies has noted that the effectiveness of primitive healers, psychotherapists, and other helping professionals depends on:

    a) the use of scientific principles
    b) the healer's experience with a wide range of problems
    c) society members' belief in the healer's power
    d) the amount of contact between the healer and the sufferer

3.60: In medicine, an example of a placebo is:

    a) a medication designed to treat a disease
    b) a test to diagnose a disorder
    c) a pill with inactive ingredients
    d) the beneficial effect of treatment

3.61: Patients in a placebo control group would:

    a) receive a treatment specifically designed for their disorder
    b) show no improvement
    c) receive no treatment, or be put on a waiting list
    d) receive a treatment not thought to be specifically effective in treating their disorder

3.62: In a double-blind study of medication:

    a) the patient doesn't know if the medication is a placebo
    b) neither the patient nor the doctor knows if the medication is a placebo
    c) there is a higher risk of expectation effects
    d) any placebo effect can be seen as a hoax

3.63: Double-blind studies of medication effectiveness are necessary because:

MC/Mod
Pg:98
kind:c
Ans:(b)

a) patients can tell if a medication is real by looking at it
b) physicians' expectations can induce a placebo effect
c) a placebo is not a treatment
d) if expectancies are too high, treatment might fail

3.64: Across different approaches to therapy, an essential element for success is:

MC/Easy
Pg:99
kind:c
Ans:(c)

a) a well developed theoretical perspective
b) not limiting goals to just a few areas
c) therapist warmth and supportiveness
d) discouragement of the therapeutic alliance

3.65: When couples therapy is used in conjunction with individual therapy:

MC/Mod
Pg:101
kind:c
Ans:(a)

a) the outcomes are often more positive
b) couples therapy interferes with individual therapy
c) individual therapy interferes with couples therapy
d) the individual improves at the couple's expense

3.66: Parent management training is designed to:

MC/Easy
Pg:102
kind:f
Ans:(d)

a) provide support for teen mothers
b) provide child care for mentally ill parents
c) educate psychiatric professionals about the demands of parenting
d) teach skills for rearing difficult children

3.67: A common goal in systems approaches to family therapy is to:

MC/Mod
Pg:102
kind:c
Ans:(d)

a) get family members to express strong emotions
b) point out how family behavior can cause psychopathology
c) train parents in behavior management
d) get the parents to cooperate as a team

3.68: Current theories of family systems therapy hold
that:

    a) family relationships and behavior cause mental
       disorders
    b) family therapy should not be used in
       conjunction with individual therapy
    c) the primary alliance in the family should be
       between parent and child
    d) troubled relationships can intensify
       psychopathology

MC/Mod
Pg:102
kind:c
Ans:(d)

3.69: Experiential group therapy places primary focus on:

    a) teaching specific information or skills
    b) bringing together people with similar problems
    c) relationships between group members
    d) a combination of research and therapy

MC/Easy
Pg:103
kind:f
Ans:(c)

3.70: Community psychology is a branch of psychology that
attempts to:

    a) expand the influence of group therapy
    b) improve individual well-being by promoting
       social change
    c) develop specific treatments for specific
       disorders
    d) promote outpatient individual therapy for
       mental disorders

MC/Easy
Pg:104
kind:f
Ans:(b)

3.71: Trying to prevent new cases of mental illness from
ever developing is called:

    a) primary prevention
    b) secondary prevention
    c) tertiary prevention
    d) social ecology

MC/Mod
Pg:104
kind:f
Ans:(a)

3.72: Efforts to detect problems early and treat them
before they get more serious are called:

    a) primary prevention
    b) secondary prevention
    c) tertiary prevention
    d) social ecology

MC/Mod
Pg:104
kind:c
Ans:(b)

3.73: Research on the effectiveness of applied
relaxation, cognitive behavioral therapy, and
nondirective therapy for treating generalized
anxiety disorder (GAD) shows that 1 year after a
12-week course of therapy:

    a) all groups were functioning equally well
    b) patients in the nondirective group were faring
       best
    c) patients in the applied relaxation group were
       faring best
    d) patients in the cognitive behavioral group were
       faring best

MC/Diff
Pg:105
kind:f
Ans:(d)

True-False Questions

3.74: The psychodynamic, behavioral, and humanistic
approaches are all forms of psychotherapy.

TF/Easy
Pg:73
kind:f
Ans:True

3.75: In behavior therapy, both the patient and the
therapist take an active role in treatment.

TF/Mod
Pg:76
kind:f
Ans:True

3.76: The scientific beginnings of the biological
treatment of mental disorders can be traced to the
19th century and the discovery of the diagnosis and
cure of general paresis.

TF/Mod
Pg:77
kind:f
Ans:True

3.77: Random assignment in an experiment ensures that
each subject has a statistically equal chance of
being assigned to a certain level of the dependent
variable.

TF/Diff
Pg:78
kind:f
Ans:False

3.78: Biological treatments for mental disorders are now
available because the specific etiology or root
cause of many mental disorders have now been
uncovered.

TF/Mod
Pg:79
kind:c
Ans:False

3.79: As practiced today, electroconvulsive therapy (ECT)
typically involves 6 or 7 administrations of
electrical current to both sides of the brain.

TF/Mod
Pg:80
kind:f
Ans:False

3.80: Tobacco and caffeine are psychoactive drugs.

TF/Easy
Pg:80
kind:f
Ans:True

3.81: The ethical standards of informed consent require that subjects be free to volunteer or to refuse to participate in research.

TF/Mod
Pg:82
kind:c
Ans:True

3.82: Psychoactive medications offer symptom relief, not a cure of underlying pathology.

TF/Mod
Pg:84
kind:c
Ans:True

3.83: The ultimate goal of psychoanalysis is to rid the patient of defense mechanisms.

TF/Mod
Pg:85
kind:c
Ans:False

3.84: Ego analysis emphasizes how a patient deals with reality and relationships.

TF/Mod
Pg:86
kind:c
Ans:True

3.85: Contingency management and token economies are based on the principle of operant conditioning.

TF/Easy
Pg:89
kind:f
Ans:True

3.86: Beck's cognitive therapy is based on attempts to get the patient to recognize irrationality based on personal conclusions rather than confrontation by the therapist.

TF/Mod
Pg:91
kind:c
Ans:True

3.87: Research on humanistic therapy has emphasized process variables such as the role of empathy in predicting successful outcomes.

TF/Diff
Pg:93
kind:c
Ans:True

3.88: Therapy outcome research shows that only about 1/3 of patients improve with therapy.

TF/Mod
Pg:95
kind:f
Ans:False

3.89: Placebos work because of an expectation that they will be effective.

TF/Easy
Pg:98
kind:c
Ans:True

3.90: An important aspect of the therapeutic process is that the therapist's interpretations decrease cognitive dissonance.

TF/Diff
Pg:100
kind:c
Ans:False

3.91: A major focus of couples therapy is to keep the marriage or relationship intact.

TF/Mod
Pg:101
kind:c
Ans:False

3.92: Group therapy is not beneficial when the patient's disorder has a clear biological cause.

TF/Mod
Pg:103
kind:c
Ans:False

3.93: Tertiary prevention is an intervention that occurs after the illness has been identified.

TF/Mod
Pg:104
kind:f
Ans:True

Essay Questions

3.94: Discuss the benefits and limitations of using experimental methods to study the etiology of abnormal behavior.

Answer: Benefit: ability to establish cause and effect through control. Limitations: practical and ethical limits to the type of variable that can be studied.

ES Moderate Page: 78 kind: c

3.95: Discuss some of the problems with using an experimental method to study various forms of psychological treatment.

Answer: Although the researcher can control random assignment to groups, the researcher cannot control drop outs, whether subjects seek additional help elsewhere, how therapy is conducted in the sessions, and whether the patient does homework or takes medication as prescribed.

ES Difficult Page: 79 kind: c

3.96: Discuss the ethical dilemmas associated with using control groups in experimental research on treatment effectiveness.

Answer: Being assigned to a control group might mean receiving no treatment. Alternatively, being in a control group might mean receiving a placebo, which may be deceptive. The patient might then be less likely to seek more appropriate treatment because they think they are being helped effectively.

ES Moderate Pages: 81-82 kind: c

3.97: Discuss the purpose of token economy systems and the limitations of token economy systems.

Answer: Purpose: apply principles of operant conditioning so that inappropriate behavior is not reinforced and appropriate behavior is reinforced with rewards or something that can be exchanged for rewards. Limitations: often use artificial rewards that would not be meaningful or available outside the treatment setting; outside the treatment setting, inappropriate behavior is often reinforced.

ES Moderate Page: 89 kind: c

3.98: In what ways is humanistic therapy different from psychodynamic and behavioral therapies? In what ways is humanistic therapy similar to psychodynamic and behavioral therapies?

Answer: Different: humanistic therapy focuses on a genuine, reciprocal relationship as the treatment, not as the means for delivering treatment. Similar to psychoanalytic: focus on uncovering hidden emotions. Similar to behavioral: focus on the present.

ES Difficult Page: 92 kind: c

3.99: Researchers have come to the general conclusion that among people with emotional problems who use therapy, about 2/3 improve. Research has also found that of people with emotional problems who do NOT use therapy, 1/3 improve, or show "spontaneous remission." There is debate about whether this figure of 1/3 is an overestimate or an underestimate of the true number of emotionally disturbed people who improve without therapy. Discuss how the definition or nature of the non-treatment group in these studies may influence this debate.

Answer: One-third may be an overestimate if many of the people who aren't in therapy are still getting treatment from other sources such as family members and pastoral counseling. One-third may be an underestimate if it is considered that even unstructured conversations with a professional can be associated with remission of problems. Finally, there may be different rates of spontaneous remission for different disorders.

ES   Difficult   Page: 95   kind: c

3.100: What factors common to all therapies are most predictive of positive outcomes?

Answer: Client expectation that therapy works; client's perception that the therapist is supportive; therapist is warm and empathic; therapist is nonjudgmental; therapist points out inconsistencies in client's thinking or behavior.

ES   Moderate   Page: 100   kind: c

Chapter 4
Classification and Assessment

Multiple Choice Questions

4.1: A psychiatric diagnosis: MC/Mod
                                                                 Pg:110
   a) explains the etiology of a problem   kind:f
   b) describes behavior as fitting the criteria for   Ans:(b)
      a specific category
   c) is based on a formulation of a treatment plan
   d) emphasizes biological, not environmental,
      contributors

4.2: The official classification system for mental   MC/Easy
     disorders used by psychologists is known as: Pg:110
                                                                 kind:f
   a) WHO   b) PDR   Ans:(c)
   c) DSM-IV   d) APA

4.3: Carolus Linnaeus is considered the "father of   MC/Easy
     taxonomy" because he: Pg:113
                                                                 kind:f
   a) developed the Library of Congress system of   Ans:(c)
      classifying books
   b) proposed dimensional rather than categorical
      classification
   c) introduced the classification system for living
      organisms
   d) delineated monothetic versus polythetic classes

4.4: The value of a classification system depends on: MC/Easy
                                                                 Pg:113
   a) the purpose for which it is developed or used   kind:c
   b) the specificity of the classification criteria   Ans:(a)
   c) the generality of the classification criteria
   d) descriptive similarities of the categories

4.5: A psychologist is classifying people in terms of   MC/Mod
     how anxious they are. If the psychologist   Pg:113
     classifies them as being either "anxious" or "not   kind:a
     anxious," she is using a classification system that   Ans:(c)
     is:

   a) dimensional   b) monothetic
   c) categorical   d) polythetic

4.6: A psychologist is classifying people in terms of
how depressed they are. The psychologist
classifies them based on their score on a
self-report measure indicating the presence of
dysphoria. A higher score indicates a higher level
of dysphoria. The psychologist is using a
classification system that is:

MC/Mod
Pg:113
kind:a
Ans:(b)

a) categorical   b) dimensional
c) monothetic   d) polythetic

4.7: If all the members of a category must possess all
the same required characteristics, the
classification system is called:

MC/Mod
Pg:114
kind:c
Ans:(d)

a) dimensional   b) categorical
c) polythetic   d) monothetic

4.8: A penguin and a robin are both considered birds,
even though they do not share all the same
characteristics. This is because the category
"bird" is:

MC/Mod
Pg:114
kind:c
Ans:(c)

a) dimensional   b) categorical
c) polythetic   d) monothetic

4.9: The discovery of the link between phenylketonuria
(PKU) and mental retardation (MR) first came about
through:

MC/Mod
Pg:114
kind:f
Ans:(d)

a) identification of a damaged chromosome
b) experimentation with eating problems in animals
c) theoretical speculation about the possible
   etiologies of MR
d) observation of intellectual deficits and
   peculiar odor in 2 MR boys

4.10: Mental disorders are currently classified on the
basis of:

MC/Easy
Pg:114
kind:c
Ans:(b)

a) biological features
b) descriptive features
c) causal mechanisms
d) theoretical relatedness

4.11: Progress toward a single, internationally accepted system of classification of mental disorders began during:

MC/Mod
Pg:115
kind:f
Ans:(c)

a) the first century B.C. in Egyptian, Greek, and Roman societies
b) the 18th century, with Linnaeus' taxonomy
c) the 19th century, with the establishment of large asylums
d) the 20th century, with the development of modern health care

4.12: Emil Kraeplin (1856-1926), a German psychiatrist, is famous for establishing:

MC/Mod
Pg:115
kind:f
Ans:(a)

a) 2 categories of psychosis
b) the International Classification of Diseases (ICD)
c) the Diagnostic and Statistical Manual of Mental Disorders (DSM)
d) a description of schizophrenia as "problems of living"

4.13: The third edition of the Diagnostic and Statistical Manual of Mental Disorders (DSM-III) made a dramatic departure from earlier classification systems because it:

MC/Mod
Pg:116
kind:c
Ans:(d)

a) included more psychoanalytic concepts
b) focused on biological etiology
c) was based on theory rather than clinical description
d) was based on detailed clinical description rather than theory

4.14: DSM-IV employs a multiaxial system of classification. This means:

MC/Easy
Pg:116
kind:f
Ans:(b)

a) classification is based on a polythetic approach
b) ratings are made of several areas of functioning
c) an individual must show all symptoms of a disorder to be diagnosed
d) it is both dimensional and categorical

4.15: Which of the following describes the multiaxial approach found in the DSM-IV?

MC/Mod
Pg:116
kind:f
Ans:(b)

a) 5 axes, 1 of which lists specific mental disorders
b) 5 axes, 2 of which list specific mental disorders
c) 3 axes, 1 of which lists specific mental disorders
d) 3 axes, 2 of which lists specific mental disorders

4.16: Labeling theory is a perspective on mental disorders that focuses on:

MC/Easy
Pg:117
kind:f
Ans:(a)

a) social factors that influence the assignment of a diagnosis
b) identification of biological causes of mental disorders
c) validity of including certain symptoms in criteria for diagnosis
d) interrater reliability in diagnosis

4.17: According to labeling theory, a psychiatric diagnosis serves to:

MC/Mod
Pg:117
kind:c
Ans:(a)

a) create a social role that perpetuates abnormal behavior
b) clarify the nature of a psychiatric disorder
c) identify etiological factors
d) eliminate bias due to social factors

4.18: In the DSM-IV, diagnoses are grouped under 18 general categories. These groupings are based on:

MC/Easy
Pg:118
kind:f
Ans:(a)

a) descriptive similarity
b) presumed causes
c) theoretical assumptions
d) biological factors

4.19: On Axis IV in the DSM-IV, psychosocial and environmental stressors are:

    a) noted if they occurred in the last year, and are relevant for treatment
    b) noted if they occurred early in life
    c) noted if they contribute to the condition, but not if they are caused by it
    d) not included in the description of stress

MC/Mod
Pg:119
kind:f
Ans:(a)

4.20: The DSM-IV is intended to:

    a) catalogue all psychiatric diagnoses since the 1800s
    b) cover problems typically seen by a mental health professional
    c) classify diagnoses based on effective treatments
    d) promote psychoanalytic concepts of diagnosis

MC/Mod
Pg:119
kind:f
Ans:(b)

4.21: Two clinical psychologists each interview and diagnose a group of patients. The extent to which the 2 psychologists agree on the diagnosis of each patient is called:

    a) reliability   b) validity
    c) utility   d) coverage

MC/Easy
Pg:121
kind:f
Ans:(a)

4.22: "Kappa" is a measure of interrater reliability that describes:

    a) the proportion of time raters agree exactly
    b) whether certain diagnoses are being disproportionately used
    c) proportion of agreement beyond chance agreement
    d) whether a clinician is equally accurate with all diagnoses

MC/Easy
Pg:121
kind:f
Ans:(c)

4.23: When we ask whether a category or diagnosis is meaningful, we are asking about its:

    a) reliability   b) coverage
    c) kappa   d) validity

MC/Easy
Pg:122
kind:f
Ans:(d)

4.24: Some psychologists have objected to the use of the DSM-IV because it is:

a) primarily controlled by physicians
b) tied to the health care system and insurance
c) theoretically biased
d) not exhaustive

MC/Mod
Pg:124
kind:f
Ans:(a)

4.25: Homosexuality is no longer listed as a psychiatric diagnosis. This change came about in the 1970s primarily because of:

a) political pressure and threatened social protest
b) low reliability in the category
c) questionable concurrent validity
d) changes in theories of the development of psychopathology

MC/Easy
Pg:125
kind:f
Ans:(a)

4.26: Many people objected to the possible diagnosis of "self-defeating personality disorder" because it:

a) was too vague to be reliably identified
b) appeared to blame victims of abuse for their problems
c) was not a valid category of true psychopathology
d) had an unknown etiology

MC/Mod
Pg:125
kind:c
Ans:(b)

4.27: In psychological assessment, an emphasis is placed on:

a) specific techniques rather than a process
b) samples of behavior from several sources or situations
c) detailed descriptions of one sample of behavior
d) predicting test results from behavior in the natural environment

MC/Mod
Pg:126
kind:c
Ans:(b)

4.28: A psychologist wants to get a measure of children's   MC/Mod
attention spans under quiet conditions. She   Pg:127
arranges for a group of children to meet   kind:a
individually with a research assistant who reads   Ans:(d)
each child a list of numbers and then asks the
child to repeat the numbers in reverse order. A
week later the children repeat this task. The
psychologist finds that the score that each child
received at week 1 and at week 2 tend to be very
similar. She concludes that this test has high:

     a) split half reliability
     b) validity
     c) interrater reliability
     d) test retest reliability

4.29: Split-half reliability is a measure of a test's: MC/Mod
                                               Pg:127
     a) internal consistency   kind:f
     b) test-retest consistency   Ans:(a)
     c) interrater consistency
     d) validity

4.30: A test is designed to assess the learning styles of   MC/Diff
preschoolers and to predict which children will   Pg:128
later show a learning disability (LD) in a regular   kind:a
school setting. An example of a false positive   Ans:(a)
would be when the test:

     a) predicts the child will show LD, but the child
        does not
     b) predicts the child will not show LD, and the
        child does
     c) shows low sensitivity
     d) shows high specificity

4.31: A psychologist administers a questionnaire about   MC/Mod
depression and suicidal ideation to a group of   Pg:128
teenagers, to detect those who may need some   kind:a
supportive counseling or therapy. A score in the   Ans:(d)
top 10% was thought to indicate a need for
treatment. An example of a false negative would be
if a teen:

     a) was not depressed but her score did not reflect
        this
     b) was not depressed and her score reflected this
     c) was depressed and her score reflected this
     d) was depressed but her score did not reflect it

4.32: An overzealous dean decides to administer a
lie-detector test to all the residents of a
dormitory, in order to find out who vandalized the
building. The lie-detector test is used to detect
liars. You are innocent of the vandalism. You
don't know who did the crime, and you don't much
care. You're just hoping the lie-detector test
doesn't point to you as a liar. You hope the
lie-detector test has:

MC/Diff
Pg:128
kind:a
Ans:(a)

   a) high specificity
   b) high sensitivity
   c) internal consistency
   d) low specificity

4.33: The main question related to sensitivity is whether
a test:

MC/Mod
Pg:128
kind:f
Ans:(a)

   a) correctly identifies all the people with a
      disorder
   b) correctly identifies all the people who do not
      have the disorder
   c) produces grossly inaccurate estimates with
      changes in sample size
   d) asks specific or broad questions

4.34: A psychologist designs a test to assess the level
of worrying and obsessive thinking shown by a group
of young adults. He believes that persons who
score high on the test are more likely to develop
obsessive-compulsive disorder (OCD). A year after
the test is administered to a group of 100 young
adults, he finds that of the 5 people he predicted
would get OCD, 4 actually developed it. He
therefore concludes that the test has:

MC/Diff
Pg:128
kind:a
Ans:(c)

   a) internal consistency
   b) specificity
   c) high predictive power
   d) low predictive power

4.35: Positive predictive power is computer using the
number of people who tested positive and eventually
developed the disorder (X), and the number of
people who tested positive and did not develop the
disorder (Y). The formula for calculating positive
predictive power is:

MC/Mod
Pg:128
kind:f
Ans:(a)

a) X / (X + Y)   b) X / Y
c) Y / X   d) (X + Y) / X

4.36: Diagnostic efficiency refers to:

MC/Easy
Pg:128
kind:f
Ans:(b)

a) the time it takes to form a diagnosis
b) the ability of a test to make correct
   predictions
c) the ability of a diagnosis to describe all of a
   patient's problems
d) the communication value in using diagnoses

4.37: The most commonly used psychological assessment
procedures are:

MC/Easy
Pg:130
kind:f
Ans:(b)

a) IQ tests   b) clinical interviews
c) personality tests d) rating scales

4.38: Clinical interviews with psychiatric patients are
important because:

MC/Easy
Pg:130
kind:c
Ans:(c)

a) diagnosis cannot be made without them
b) they incorporate talk therapy
c) many psychiatric symptoms are subjective
d) the therapist can explain the diagnosis

4.39: Researchers conducting epidemiological studies
often employ structured interviews because they:

MC/Mod
Pg:131
kind:c
Ans:(a)

a) increase the reliability of diagnostic
   decisions
b) increase the validity of diagnostic decisions
c) reduce the need to establish rapport
d) reduce the need for clinical judgment

4.40: A disadvantage of structured clinical interviews is that:

MC/Easy
Pg:132
kind:c
Ans:(d)

a) there is no room for clinical judgment
b) they are based only on open-ended questions
c) the interviewer cannot control the course of the interview
d) information provided by the client can be distorted

4.41: Rating scales:

MC/Easy
Pg:133
kind:c
Ans:(c)

a) record the frequency of specific behaviors
b) produce qualitative descriptions
c) provide abstract descriptions, requiring social judgments
d) are not affected by the observer's clinical experience

4.42: Compared to rating scales, behavioral coding systems:

MC/Mod
Pg:133
kind:c
Ans:(b)

a) are less reliable
b) require less inference by the observer
c) are more qualitative
d) are less affected by clinical experience

4.43: Self-monitoring refers to:

MC/Easy
Pg:134
kind:f
Ans:(d)

a) clinicians looking out for their own biases
b) the importance of the clinician's presence in formal observation
c) children learning to regulate their own behavior
d) adult clients keeping records of their own behavior

4.44: Reactivity refers to:

MC/Easy
Pg:135
kind:f
Ans:(b)

a) personal judgment affecting observers' ratings
b) a person changing her behavior when she knows she being is observed
c) the tendency for observers to rate less severity over time
d) the tendency for a person to reveal less in a structured interview than on a questionnaire

4.45: The benefit of personality tests in psychological assessment is that:

    a) it is more useful to assess personality than specific behaviors
    b) they don't have to be administered and interpreted by trained clinicians
    c) people are generally unable to describe their own personalities
    d) the same stimuli are used every time the test is given

MC/Easy
Pg:135
kind:c
Ans:(d)

4.46: Scoring of the MMPI:

    a) is objective
    b) is subjective
    c) is based on rating scales of behaviors and symptoms
    d) depends on whether the person is considered normal or pathological

MC/Easy
Pg:136
kind:f
Ans:(a)

4.47: The validity scales of the MMPI:

    a) allow comparison between observers' ratings and patient ratings
    b) reflect the patient's consistency and attitude toward the test
    c) ask about previous and current psychiatric diagnoses
    d) are used today to double check patient identification

MC/Mod
Pg:136
kind:f
Ans:(b)

4.48: An actuarial procedure of interpretation of psychological tests relies on:

    a) current behavior rather than past behavior
    b) psychoanalytic interpretation of test results
    c) subjective ratings of clinical interviews
    d) probability statements derived from empirical research

MC/Mod
Pg:136
kind:f
Ans:(d)

4.49: One of the limitations of the MMPI as a personality measure is:

    a) that it is based largely on diagnostic concepts from the 1940s
    b) that scoring is subjective
    c) its use is limited to normal personality
    d) that there is not much research on its reliability or validity

MC/Mod
Pg:138
kind:f
Ans:(a)

4.50: Projective personality tests were designed with the assumption that:

    a) a person's goals for the future tell a lot about personality
    b) visual processing errors may indicate schizophrenia
    c) self-report checklists would be more efficient than interviews
    d) individuals would project unconscious feelings onto ambiguous stimuli

MC/Easy
Pg:139
kind:c
Ans:(d)

4.51: A widely accepted approach to identifying cases of depression depends on the use of structured interviews in combination with specific diagnostic criteria listed in the DSM-IV. One problem with this procedure is that:

    a) the resulting diagnoses are not particularly reliable
    b) the resulting diagnoses are frequently not valid
    c) the approach is expensive and time-consuming
    d) the diagnoses are not made by trained clinicians

MC/Mod
Pg:140
kind:c
Ans:(c)

4.52: One problem associated with self-report measures such as the Beck Depression Inventory (BDI) is that:

    a) they are not very efficient
    b) the same information can be gained from observation
    c) they are inappropriately used for diagnostic purposes
    d) they are not very useful for research

MC/Mod
Pg:141
kind:c
Ans:(c)

4.53: The Beck Depression Inventory is most useful as:

    a) a diagnostic indicator of the presence of
       depression
    b) an index of severity of depression
    c) a structured interview
    d) a projective test

4.54: As originally designed, the Rorschach was scored
based on:

    a) the way descriptions take into account shapes
       and colors
    b) how verbally expressive the patient was
    c) psychoanalytic interpretation of the symbolism
       and content of the person's responses
    d) the emotions expressed by patients looking at
       the cards

4.55: An objective scoring system for the Rorschach was
devised by Exner in the 1980s. This scoring system
is based on:

    a) psychoanalytic interpretation of responses'
       symbolism and content
    b) the way descriptions take into account shapes
       and colors
    c) how verbally expressive the response was
    d) the emotions expressed by patients looking at
       the cards

4.56: The main advantage of projective personality tests
over other forms of personality tests is:

    a) that they may help reluctant patients express
       themselves
    b) objective scoring
    c) extensive research on validity
    d) self-administration is efficient

4.57: A measure of one aspect of a patient's social
system is the Camberwell Family Interview (CFI),
which assesses expressed emotion. Expressed
emotion is:

MC/Mod
Pg:143
kind:f
Ans:(c)

a) the patient's range of affect and mood
b) attachment between therapist and patient
c) family members' hostility toward and criticism
of the patient
d) support provided by the patient's social
network

4.58: The Family Interaction Coding System (FICS) is:

MC/Mod
Pg:143
kind:f
Ans:(d)

a) a self-report measure of family relationships
b) an interview for assessing expressed emotion
c) an assessment tool that is not associated with
reactivity
d) a reliable observational measure

4.59: Which of the following is true about the autonomic
nervous system?

MC/Easy
Pg:144
kind:f
Ans:(a)

a) responsible for body processes outside
conscious awareness
b) regulates voluntary muscle movements
c) communicates between brain and external sense
receptors
d) part of the central nervous system

4.60: The biological system that is highly reactive to
environmental events, and that can provide useful
information regarding a person's emotional states,
is:

MC/Easy
Pg:144
kind:f
Ans:(c)

a) the central nervous system
b) the somatic nervous system
c) the autonomic nervous system
d) the brain stem

4.61: Penile and vaginal plethysmographs are used to:

MC/Mod
Pg:145
kind:f
Ans:(c)

a) induce arousal in cases of sexual dysfunction
b) track brain wave activity during sexual arousal
c) measure physiological changes in the genitals
and reflect levels of sexual arousal
d) assess the association between REM sleep and
sexual activity

4.62: One purpose of physiological assessment is to
      identify meaningful subtypes of mental disorder.
      Which of the following has been found to be
      associated with a poor response to treatment for
      depression?

MC/Diff
Pg:145
kind:c
Ans:(d)

    a) impaired eye tracking
    b) high reactivity in heart rate
    c) poor response to the penile plethysmograph
    d) rapid onset of REM sleep

4.63: Sometimes physiological data provide additional
      information not available through observation. In
      research on marital relationships, an example of
      this is that in laboratory studies, dissatisfied
      husbands:

MC/Diff
Pg:146
kind:c
Ans:(b)

    a) show low physiological arousal
    b) show high arousal but do not express it
    c) show the same arousal as satisfied husbands
    d) show the same arousal as their wives

4.64: A limitation of the use of physiological assessment
      is that:

MC/Easy
Pg:146
kind:c
Ans:(d)

    a) there is very little variability in people's
       physiological reactions
    b) they provide little information beyond what
       patients can report themselves
    c) there is a high correlation among different
       autonomic response systems
    d) there is a low correlation among different
       autonomic response systems

4.65: One recent application of brain imaging techniques
      is to:

MC/Mod
Pg:146
kind:c
Ans:(a)

    a) create dynamic images of the brain while the
       person performs different tasks
    b) assess personality using projective techniques
    c) measure physiological changes in the genitalia
       associated with sexual arousal
    d) test the association between imagination and
       EEG patterns

4.66: A CT scan of the brain uses: MC/Diff
                                                            Pg:146
    a) magnetic resonance to measure photon activity   kind:f
    b) X-rays to measure photon activity   Ans:(d)
    c) magnetic resonance to measure tissue density
    d) X-rays to measure tissue density

True-False Questions

4.67: A categorical classification system assumes that   TF/Easy
      there are qualitative differences between members   Pg:113
      of different categories.   kind:c
                                                            Ans:True

4.68: Phenylketonuria (PKU) is an inherited metabolic   TF/Easy
      disorder which can cause mental retardation.   Pg:114
                                                            kind:f
                                                            Ans:True

4.69: The Diagnostic and Statistical Manual (DSM) was   TF/Easy
      designed because the International Classification   Pg:116
      of Diseases (ICD) does not include mental   kind:f
      disorders.   Ans:False

4.70: The DSM-IV is published by the American   TF/Easy
      Psychological Association.   Pg:116
                                                            kind:f
                                                            Ans:False

4.71: In the DSM-IV, Axis I and Axis II were   TF/Mod
      distinguished in order to draw attention to   Pg:118
      conditions such as personality disorder, which   kind:c
      might be overlooked in the presence of more   Ans:True
      dramatic clinical syndromes.

4.72: The question of whether a disorder runs in families   TF/Diff
      through genetic inheritance is related to the issue   Pg:123
      of predictive validity.   kind:f
                                                            Ans:False

4.73: The clinician's choice of the level of analysis   TF/Easy
      will determine in large part the assessment   Pg:126
      instruments used.   kind:c
                                                            Ans:True

76

4.74: Whether a test will pick up or detect all the cases of schizophrenia among a group of homeless persons is a question of the test's specificity.

TF/Mod
Pg:128
kind:f
Ans:False

4.75: The only diagnostic category in DSM-IV that is defined in terms of a psychological test score is mental retardation.

TF/Easy
Pg:130
kind:f
Ans:True

4.76: Most of the categories defined in DSM-IV require psychological testing in order to make a diagnosis.

TF/Mod
Pg:130
kind:f
Ans:False

4.77: Informal observations produce primarily qualitative descriptions of behavior.

TF/Easy
Pg:132
kind:f
Ans:True

4.78: Behavioral coding systems are primarily useful as an overall index of symptom severity or functional impairment.

TF/Diff
Pg:133
kind:f
Ans:False

4.79: One disadvantage of projective tests is low reliability of scoring and interpretation.

TF/Easy
Pg:143
kind:f
Ans:True

4.80: Assessments of the effects of biological systems on behavior are seldom used for the diagnosis of psychopathology in clinical practice.

TF/Easy
Pg:144
kind:f
Ans:True

4.81: One purpose of physiological assessment procedures is the identification of meaningful subtypes of mental disorders.

TF/Easy
Pg:145
kind:f
Ans:True

4.82: One of the uses of measuring regional cerebral blood flow (rCBF) is to track cerebral blood flow during certain tasks, such as blood flow to the visual cortex during visual stimulation.

TF/Easy
Pg:147
kind:f
Ans:True

4.83: One limitation of brain imaging techniques in the   TF/Easy
diagnosis of psychopathology is the lack of   Pg:147
information about norms--that is, data about   kind:f
"average" or expected results on these tests.   Ans:True

Essay Questions

4.84: What are two main uses of a classification system for abnormal behavior?

Answer: (1) matching clients' problems with the most effective treatment
(2) search for knowledge, and the possibility of identifying unique disorders so that treatments can later be developed

ES   Moderate   Page: 115   kind: c

4.85: During the 1950s and 1960s, psychiatric classification systems were widely criticized. Discuss some of the reasons for this criticism.

Answer: (1) empirical: low reliability and interrater consistency
(2) the idea that people who are diagnosed as mentally ill actually are having "problems in living"
(3) the problem of self-fulfilling prophecies: those who are diagnosed live up to the expectations of the "sick" role

ES   Moderate   Page: 116   kind: c

4.86: Describe the different ways in which diagnosis can be useful or valid.

Answer: (1) meaningful or important: provides information and communication value
(2) etiological: provides information on cause
(3) concurrent: agrees with information about behavior in other situations and from other sources
(4) predictive: provides information about the predictable course of the disorder, and later status and behavior

ES   Moderate   Page: 123   kind: c

78

4.87: Describe the 3 primary goals of psychological assessment, and give an example of each.

Answer: (1) predictions: Will this person engage in violence if he is released from jail?
(2) plan interventions: Does this person have the intelligence level necessary to benefit from insight-oriented therapy?
(3) evaluate treatment effectiveness: Has this person's depression decreased over the course of therapy?

ES Difficult Page: 126 kind: c

4.88: Describe a case where it would be better to have high specificity, even at the cost of lower sensitivity. Describe a case where it would be better to have high sensitivity, even at the cost of specificity.

Answer: (1) High specificity would be desired in the case of accusing someone of a crime; one would not want to falsely accuse or prosecute an innocent person.
(2) High sensitivity would be desired in the case of testing people for exposure to radiation so that they can be treated. In this case it would be harmful to miss someone who actually had been exposed to radiation and who therefore would not be treated.

ES Moderate Page: 128 kind: c

4.89: A researcher wants to measure patients' anxiety while discussing upcoming feared events. She measures heart rate before, during, and after a patient's discussion. She finds that discussion of the upcoming feared event is associated with increased heart rate, and concludes that such discussions are associated with increased anxiety. Discuss the grounds on which such a conclusion would be criticized.

Answer: (1) Physiological assessment is not sufficient, and the measurement of anxiety should include self-report.
(2) Any individual autonomic response has low correlation with other autonomic responses. Had the researcher measured perspiration, for example, she might have drawn a different conclusion. Several different physiological measures should be used. (3) Reactivity and stability vary from individual to individual. For some, anxiety may be associated with great increases in heart rate; for others, anxiety may be associated with small increases in heart rate. (4) The increased heart rate could be due to person variables (the nature of her sample) or to situational variables (such as having to discuss anything in front of a stranger).

ES Difficult Page: 144 kind: c

Chapter 5
Mood Disorders

Multiple Choice Questions

5.1: Affect refers to:

    a) observable behaviors associated with subjective
       feelings
    b) subjective feelings
    c) a state of arousal
    d) physiological changes associated with
       subjective feelings

MC/Mod
Pg:152
kind:f
Ans:(a)

5.2: Which of the following is an example of expression
    of affect?

    a) your heart rate increases
    b) your face shows a grimace
    c) you say you feel angry
    d) you beat someone up

MC/Mod
Pg:152
kind:a
Ans:(b)

5.3: One of the features of mania is:

    a) schizophrenic behaviors
    b) elated mood
    c) criminality
    d) blunted affect

MC/Easy
Pg:152
kind:f
Ans:(b)

5.4: Mary Beth has had two episodes of major depression
    and no other periods of psychological disturbance.
    Which label best describes her condition?

    a) unipolar mood disorder
    b) bipolar mood disorder
    c) double depression
    d) dysthymia

MC/Mod
Pg:153
kind:a
Ans:(a)

5.5: Robert has had one episode of mania. Which label
    best describes his condition?

    a) bipolar mood disorder
    b) unipolar mood disorder
    c) dysthymia
    d) dysphoric mood disorder

MC/Mod
Pg:153
kind:a
Ans:(a)

5.6: Dysphoria is:

    a) depressed mood
    b) elated mood
    c) inappropriate affect
    d) labile affect

MC/Mod
Pg:155
kind:f
Ans:(a)

5.7: Euphoria is characterized by:

    a) depressed mood
    b) inappropriate affect
    c) elated mood
    d) labile affect

MC/Mod
Pg:155
kind:f
Ans:(c)

5.8: The depressive triad refers to:

    a) attention to negative features of the self, environment, future
    b) emotional, behavioral, and cognitive changes in depression
    c) major depression, dysphoria, and double depression
    d) unipolar mood disorder, bipolar I disorder, and bipolar II disorder

MC/Mod
Pg:156
kind:f
Ans:(a)

5.9: Betsy believes she is less capable than her co-workers, even though she has won many awards for her performance. She often feels lonely and believes no one wants to be her friend. Her future seems empty and meaningless to her. These traits characterize:

    a) information processing deficits in depression
    b) the "depressive triad"
    c) neurotic depression
    d) dysthymia

MC/Mod
Pg:156
kind:a
Ans:(b)

5.10: One symptom that a person with mania and a person with depression may have in common is:

    a) thoughts slowing down
    b) being easily distracted
    c) feelings of worthlessness
    d) oversleeping

MC/Diff
Pg:156
kind:c
Ans:(b)

5.11: An example of a somatic or vegetative symptom of   MC/Mod
       depression is: Pg:157
                                                               kind:f
       a) pessimistic thoughts about the future   Ans:(c)
       b) feelings of low self-worth
       c) sleeping problems
       d) suicidality

5.12: Psychomotor retardation, characterized by slowed   MC/Mod
       speech and movements, is: Pg:157
                                                               kind:c
       a) a symptom of clinical depression   Ans:(a)
       b) a side effect of many antidepressant
          medications
       c) a vulnerability factor for depression
       d) part of the depressive triad

5.13: Somatic symptoms are also known as: MC/Mod
                                                               Pg:157
       a) depressive   b) neurological   kind:f
       c) unipolar   d) vegetative   Ans:(d)

5.14: The emotion which is thought to be most important   MC/Diff
       in predicting suicide is: Pg:158
                                                               kind:c
       a) depressed feelings   b) hopelessness   Ans:(b)
       c) anger   d) anxiety

5.15: Comorbidity refers to: MC/Mod
                                                               Pg:159
       a) death as a consequence of suicide   kind:f
       b) symptoms of more than one underlying disorder   Ans:(b)
       c) death related to mental disorder
       d) a tendency for mental illness to run in
          families

5.16: Whose name is associated with the early   MC/Mod
       classification of mental disorder in terms of the   Pg:160
       categories of dementia praecox and manic depressive   kind:f
       psychosis?   Ans:(d)

       a) Beck   b) Freud
       c) Lewinsohn   d) Kraeplin

82

5.17: In contrast to Kraeplin's system of classification of mental disorder, the classification system of psychiatrists such as Meyer and Freud places greater emphasis on:

MC/Diff
Pg:160
kind:c
Ans:(d)

  a) more serious forms of mental disorder
  b) dementia praecox and manic depressive psychosis
  c) the role of biological factors in etiology
  d) the role of environmental events in etiology

5.18: One important consideration in distinguishing clinical depression from normal sadness is that clinical depression:

MC/Mod
Pg:160
kind:c
Ans:(c)

  a) is caused by an identifiable precipitant
  b) occurs only in people who suffered early losses
  c) is accompanied by difficulties in concentration, eating, and sleep
  d) involves changes in brain chemistry

5.19: One piece of evidence suggesting that unipolar and bipolar mood disorders may be distinct disorders is that:

MC/Mod
Pg:161
kind:c
Ans:(a)

  a) bipolar disorder has a younger average age of onset
  b) genetic factors are more influential for unipolar mood disorder
  c) unipolar mood disorder responds to lithium carbonate
  d) people with mania usually don't also have depression

5.20: The difference between Bipolar I and Bipolar II is that:

MC/Mod
Pg:161
kind:f
Ans:(b)

  a) Bipolar I involves hypomania, not mania
  b) Bipolar II involves hypomania, not mania
  c) Bipolar I responds to lithium carbonate
  d) Bipolar II responds to lithium carbonate

5.21: Which is the most typical course of unipolar mood disorder?

MC/Mod
Pg:161
kind:c
Ans:(d)

  a) a single episode of major depression
  b) cycling episodes of depression and mania
  c) a single episode of mania
  d) several episodes of major depression

5.22: One way that dysthymia differs from major
      depression is that it:

    a) usually lasts longer
    b) responds better to medication
    c) is more severe
    d) usually has a precipitating event

MC/Mod
Pg:161
kind:c
Ans:(a)

5.23: Hypomania is an episode:

    a) of high energy, but less severe than mania
    b) of high energy, but more severe than mania
    c) occurring during the depressed phase of bipolar
       illness
    d) characterizing Bipolar I and Bipolar II but not
       cyclothymia

MC/Mod
Pg:162
kind:c
Ans:(a)

5.24: A chronic but less severe form of bipolar disorder
      is:

    a) unipolar disorder   b) dysthymia
    c) hypomania   d) cyclothymia

MC/Mod
Pg:163
kind:f
Ans:(d)

5.25: Melancholia is a term for:

    a) dysthymia
    b) a particularly severe type of depression
    c) neurotic depression
    d) normal sadness unrelated to clinical depression

MC/Mod
Pg:163
kind:f
Ans:(b)

5.26: The most typical seasonal pattern in mood disorders
      is:

    a) depression in summer
    b) depression in winter
    c) mania in summer
    d) mania in winter

MC/Easy
Pg:163
kind:f
Ans:(b)

5.27: Rapid cycling bipolar disorder is characterized by:

    a) development of a manic episode in less than a
       week
    b) many mood shifts per day
    c) about four cycles of depression and mania per
       year
    d) a seasonal pattern of symptoms

MC/Diff
Pg:163
kind:f
Ans:(c)

5.28: Other than the presence of manic episodes in bipolar mood disorder, the main distinguishing factor between unipolar and bipolar mood disorders is:

MC/Diff
Pg:164
kind:c
Ans:(a)

   a) earlier onset and worse prognosis in bipolar mood disorder
   b) earlier onset and better prognosis in bipolar mood disorder
   c) later onset and worse prognosis in bipolar mood disorder
   d) later onset and better prognosis in bipolar mood disorder

5.29: The average number of depressive episodes in unipolar mood disorder is:

MC/Mod
Pg:164
kind:f
Ans:(b)

   a) 1-2   b) 5-6
   c) 8-10   d) 15 or more

5.30: Point prevalence of depression refers to the percentage of the population that:

MC/Mod
Pg:165
kind:f
Ans:(d)

   a) can be expected to experience depression at some point in their life
   b) report at least one symptom of depression over the last year
   c) have developed depression for the first time during the past year
   d) report being depressed at one given point in time

5.31: According to the Epidemiological Catchment Area (ECA) study, what percentage of people (men and women) in the U.S. can be expected to be affected by depression at any given point in time?

MC/Mod
Pg:165
kind:f
Ans:(c)

   a) 1-2%   b) 5-8%
   c) 13-20%   d) 40-50%

5.32: Cross-cultural studies of psychopathology suggest that:

    a) DSM categories are culture-free
    b) Chinese psychiatrists often mistake depression and anxiety for neurasthenia
    c) depression, anxiety, and associated somatic complaints are universal psychological phenomena
    d) there are very different rates of mood disorder in western and nonwestern countries

MC/Diff
Pg:167
kind:c
Ans:(c)

5.33: Large-scale cross-cultural studies have shown that compared to European cultures, non-European cultures have higher rates of which symptom of depression?

    a) somatization   b) guilt feelings
    c) suicidal ideation   d) sleep disturbances

MC/Mod
Pg:167
kind:f
Ans:(a)

5.34: Cross-cultural studies have found that neurasthenia (typified by loss of energy, dizziness, loss of appetite, poor concentration, nightmares) is commonly diagnosed in China but rarely diagnosed in Western societies. This is because:

    a) these symptoms are much more common in China
    b) these symptoms are classified as depression and anxiety in the U.S.
    c) the Chinese psychiatrists use outdated procedures
    d) Western psychiatry places less emphasis on physical symptoms

MC/Mod
Pg:167
kind:c
Ans:(b)

5.35: Since the 1960s, rates of suicide have increased most among:

    a) the elderly   b) the middle aged
    c) adolescents   d) children

MC/Mod
Pg:168
kind:f
Ans:(c)

5.36: Freud's view of depression focused on:

    a) the lack of positive emotions in early relationships
    b) the parents' narcissistic involvement with the child
    c) the patient's irrational self-criticism
    d) the depressed person's anger at someone they had lost

MC/Diff
Pg:170
kind:c
Ans:(d)

5.37: According to Freud, people who are predisposed to
       depression tend to form "narcissistic"
       relationships. This means:

    a) they express only negative feelings toward
       people who are close to them
    b) their relationships are emotionally shallow,
       with few strong feelings
    c) they depend on the other person to maintain
       their self-esteem
    d) they alienate others because of their
       ambivalence

MC/Diff
Pg:170
kind:c
Ans:(c)

5.38: The number of stressful events experienced by
       depressed persons is:

    a) lower than average
    b) comparable to that experienced by the average
       person
    c) higher than average
    d) unrelated to the onset of depression

MC/Mod
Pg:171
kind:c
Ans:(c)

5.39: In their study of the link between depression and
       stressful life events, Brown and Harris studied a
       sample of women who were considered to be at
       especially high risk for depression. This sample
       was characterized by being:

    a) ages 18-50 with children living at home
    b) widowed
    c) unmarried and working
    d) women whose own mothers were depressed

MC/Mod
Pg:172
kind:c
Ans:(a)

5.40: Brown and Harris followed women over a one-year
       period to study the link between depression and
       stressful life events. They found that:

    a) of those who became depressed, only a few had
       experienced a severe life event
    b) of those who became depressed, most had
       experienced a severe life event
    c) of those who experienced a severe life event,
       most became depressed
    d) of those who experienced a severe life event,
       few became depressed

MC/Diff
Pg:172
kind:c
Ans:(b)

5.41: Prospective research by Brown and Harris on the   MC/Diff
       development of depression in women with young   Pg:173
       children found that the likelihood of a woman   kind:c
       becoming depressed was especially high if she   Ans:(b)
       experienced a loss or stressful event in an area of
       her life:

       a) in which she had not previously had
          difficulties
       b) in which she was already experiencing
          difficulties
       c) about which she was not confident
       d) about which she was confident

5.42: Which of the following was a characteristic that   MC/Mod
       Brown and Harris found increased a woman's chances   Pg:173
       of becoming depressed if she experienced a severe   kind:c
       life event?   Ans:(b)

       a) a conflictual marriage
       b) having several young children at home
       c) working outside the house
       d) a poor relationship with her own mother

5.43: According to Beck, which of the following is an   MC/Mod
       example of a cognitive distortion typical of   Pg:174
       depression?   kind:c
                                                                Ans:(c)
       a) turning anger at others toward the self
       b) inability to concentrate
       c) selectively remembering more negative events
          than positive events
       d) suicidal ideation

5.44: A schema is: MC/Mod
                                                                Pg:174
       a) a point of contention or conflict in a   kind:f
          relationship   Ans:(d)
       b) a role played in a relationship
       c) an example of a cognitive distortion
       d) an organized cognitive representation of prior
          experiences

5.45: The learned helplessness theory of depression was developed based on studies of rats exposed to the stress of being shocked. Which of the following behaviors was thought to provide a model of depression?

MC/Mod
Pg:175
kind:c
Ans:(c)

    a) aggressiveness in response to inescapable shock
    b) aggressiveness in response to controllable shock
    c) passivity in response to inescapable shock
    d) passivity in response to controllable shock

5.46: The hopelessness theory of depression holds that depressed persons:

MC/Diff
Pg:175
kind:c
Ans:(d)

    a) have a pessimistic view that only bad things will happen
    b) make external causal attributions
    c) make unstable causal attributions
    d) believe that things happen regardless of what the person does

5.47: Mary Ellen fails a calculus exam. Although other students who failed the same exam complain that the exam was too hard and the professor has a reputation for tough grading, Mary Ellen is convinced that she failed the exam because she is incapable of understanding the material covered on the exam. This is an example of a "depressogenic" attribution style that is:

MC/Diff
Pg:175
kind:a
Ans:(a)

    a) internal   b) global
    c) stable   d) causal

5.48: Robert strikes out during a softball game, causing his team to lose the game. He begins to brood about his failure, and concludes that not only is he a failure in sports, but in all areas of his life. This is an example of a "depressogenic" attribution style which is:

MC/Diff
Pg:175
kind:a
Ans:(c)

    a) internal   b) stable
    c) global   d) causal

89

5.49: Lewinsohn's behavioral model views reduced activity level and withdrawal typical of depression as related to:

MC/Mod
Pg:175
kind:c
Ans:(b)

    a) increases in positive reinforcement
    b) reductions in positive reinforcement
    c) increases in negative reinforcement
    d) reductions in negative reinforcement

5.50: Meredith is depressed. According to Coyne's interpersonal view of depression, which is a likely description of Meredith?

MC/Mod
Pg:176
kind:a
Ans:(a)

    a) her interpersonal style may annoy others
    b) she erroneously believes that her relationships are inadequate
    c) she has not resolved grief over early childhood losses
    d) she makes internal causal attributions

5.51: Some research evidence suggests that persons who show a ruminative style by writing in a diary or talking extensively with a friend about their depressed mood show:

MC/Mod
Pg:176
kind:c
Ans:(d)

    a) shorter and less severe depressed mood
    b) increased empathy
    c) good ability to distract themselves from their bad mood
    d) longer and more severe depressed mood

5.52: Bill's girlfriend breaks up with him and he interprets this as a sign that he is a worthless person. He then becomes depressed. The cause of his depression is best conceptualized as:

MC/Mod
Pg:177
kind:a
Ans:(c)

    a) the loss of the interpersonal relationship
    b) the cognitive interpretation of the loss
    c) the interaction of interpersonal and cognitive factors
    d) biological factors unrelated to these events

90

5.53: Women's higher vulnerability to depression is
sometimes interpreted to be the result of gender
differences in how men and women interpret
interpersonal events. Specifically, when something
bad happens to a friend or family member, women
tend to:

    a) blame themselves for what happened
    b) avoid thinking about practical solutions
    c) interpret the situation as worse than it is
    d) experience it as if it were happening to them

MC/Mod
Pg:177
kind:c
Ans:(d)

5.54: In research on familial patterns of mood disorders,
the proband is:

    a) the percentage of family members showing the
       mood disorder
    b) the specific mood disorder being studied
    c) a twin who does not show the mood disorder
    d) a family member identified as having a mood
       disorder

MC/Mod
Pg:178
kind:f
Ans:(d)

5.55: Among family members of a depressed person with
unipolar mood disorder, the rate of bipolar mood
disorder is:

    a) significantly lower than in the general
       population
    b) significantly higher than in the general
       population
    c) about the same as in the general population
    d) similar to rates of unipolar in the general
       population

MC/Diff
Pg:178
kind:f
Ans:(c)

5.56: Studies of the concordance rates for unipolar mood
disorder and bipolar mood disorder in monozygotic
(MZ) and dizygotic (DZ) twins suggest:

    a) a larger role of genetic factors in bipolar
       mood disorder
    b) a larger role of genetic factors in unipolar
       mood disorder
    c) similar concordance rates for unipolar mood
       disorder in MZ and DZ twins
    d) similar concordance rates for bipolar mood
       disorder in MZ and DZ twins

MC/Mod
Pg:179
kind:f
Ans:(a)

5.57: Which of the following is evidence that
environmental factors mediate the expression of a
genetically determined vulnerability to depression?

MC/Diff
Pg:179
kind:c
Ans:(b)

    a) concordance rates for MZ twins are greater than
for DZ twins

    b) concordance rates for MZ twins are less than
100%

    c) concordance rates for MZ twins and DZ twins are
the same

    d) concordance rates for MZ twins are less than
for DZ twins

5.58: Environmental factors seem to account for the
highest proportion of variance in which of the
following disorders?

MC/Diff
Pg:179
kind:c
Ans:(a)

    a) dysthymia   b) bipolar disorder

    c) unipolar disorder   d) cyclothymia

5.59: In research on the heritability of mood disorders,
linkage studies examine:

MC/Mod
Pg:180
kind:c
Ans:(b)

    a) rates of mood disorder in MZ and DZ twins

    b) the association between a mood disorder and
another trait within the same family

    c) rates of mood disorder in children of depressed
probands

    d) the effects of medication on symptoms

5.60: Serotonin and norepinephrine are known as:

MC/Mod
Pg:180
kind:f
Ans:(a)

    a) monoamines   b) tricyclics

    c) MAO inhibitors   d) antidepressants

5.61: The indolamine hypothesis of depression held that:

MC/Mod
Pg:181
kind:c
Ans:(d)

    a) mania is associated with lower levels of
norepinephrine

    b) depression is associated with lower levels of
norepinephrine

    c) mania is associated with higher levels of
serotonin

    d) depression is associated with higher levels of
serotonin

5.62: The most recent theories of the neurophysiology of   MC/Diff
depression focus on the role of: Pg:181
                                                            kind:c

    a) the sensitivity and density of postsynaptic   Ans:(a)
       receptors

    b) the amount of dopamine available in the
       presynaptic neuron

    c) the amount of serotonin present in the synapse

    d) the rate of production of norepinephrine

5.63: Early evidence for the role of hormones in the   MC/Diff
etiology of depression came from studies of   Pg:181
patients with Cushing's disease. What characterized   kind:c
these patients?   Ans:(b)

    a) high depression with low cortisol

    b) high depression with high cortisol

    c) mania with low cortisol

    d) mania with high cortisol

5.64: Failure to suppress production of the natural   MC/Mod
hormone cortisol in response to the dexamethasone   Pg:182
suppression test suggests a dysfunction in which   kind:f
system in the etiology of depression?   Ans:(b)

    a) neurotransmitter system

    b) hypothalamus-pituitary-adrenal axis

    c) genetics

    d) MAO inhibition

5.65: Research on the interaction of biological and   MC/Diff
psychological factors in producing depression has   Pg:182
been conducted using studies of animals' responses   kind:c
to stress. Specifically, research by Jay Weiss has   Ans:(c)
found that whether rats exposed to uncontrollable
shock react with "depressed" behavior depends on:

    a) the number of shocks, independent of brain
       chemistry changes

    b) the level of norepinephrine, independent of the
       number of shocks

    c) whether the stress causes drops in brain
       norepinephrine

    d) whether the stress causes increases in brain
       norepinephrine

5.66: Analogue studies: MC/Mod
                                                           Pg:183
   a) focus on behaviors that resemble mental   kind:c
      disorders   Ans:(a)
   b) study mental disorders in the natural
      environment
   c) examine rates of mental illness in families of
      patients
   d) focus on surgical techniques with animals

5.67: The primary advantage of analogue studies in   MC/Mod
      research on mood disorders is that they: Pg:183
                                                           kind:c
   a) can use animals rather than humans   Ans:(c)
   b) are not subject to Ethics Review Boards
   c) can employ an experimental procedure
   d) are highly generalizable to situations outside
      the laboratory

5.68: Which of the following typifies a cognitive therapy MC/Mod
      approach to the treatment of depression?   Pg:184
                                                           kind:c
   a) probing for unconscious roots of anger   Ans:(c)
   b) focusing on early childhood experiences
   c) reducing patients' self-defeating thoughts
   d) increasing internal causal attributions

5.69: Interpersonal therapy for depression focuses on: MC/Mod
                                                           Pg:185
   a) unconscious feelings for the attachment figure   kind:c
   b) close, dependent relationship with the   Ans:(d)
      therapist
   c) patterns learned in childhood relationships
   d) current relationship difficulties

5.70: The Treatment of Depression Collaborative Research   MC/Diff
      Program compared the effectiveness of cognitive,   Pg:185
      interpersonal, and drug therapies. At a very   kind:c
      general level, the results indicated that: Ans:(d)

   a) cognitive therapy was most effective
   b) interpersonal therapy was most effective
   c) drug therapy was most effective
   d) all three treatments were equally effective

5.71: The Treatment of Depression Collaborative Research
       Program compared the effectiveness of cognitive,
       interpersonal, and drug therapies. At the 18 month
       followup:

       a) patients in the three active groups were still
          doing better than the control group
       b) patients in the three active groups were no
          longer doing better than the control group
       c) only the medication group was still doing
          better
       d) only the medication group was doing worse

MC/Diff
Pg:186
kind:c
Ans:(b)

5.72: The use of electroconvulsive therapy (ECT) in
       treating severe depression:

       a) is minimally effective
       b) can be more effective than antidepressant
          medication
       c) is no longer practiced in the U.S.
       d) typically requires many months of
          administration

MC/Mod
Pg:186
kind:c
Ans:(b)

5.73: One of the possible side effects of
       electroconvulsive therapy (ECT) is:

       a) weight gain   b) memory impairment
       c) anxiety   d) fatigue

MC/Easy
Pg:186
kind:f
Ans:(b)

5.74: Tricyclic drugs produce their antidepressant effect
       by:

       a) blocking production of norepinephrine and
          dopamine
       b) increasing production of norepinephrine and
          dopamine
       c) blocking reuptake of norepinephrine and
          dopamine
       d) increasing reuptake of norepinephrine and
          dopamine

MC/Diff
Pg:187
kind:c
Ans:(c)

5.75: One of the reasons MAO inhibitors aren't used as frequently as tricyclics is:

    a) their higher cost
    b) a slower reaction rate
    c) they produce high blood pressure if patient eats foods containing tyramine
    d) side effect of abnormal EEG

MC/Diff
Pg:187
kind:c
Ans:(c)

5.76: In contrast to MAO inhibitors and tricyclics, the selective serotonin reuptake inhibitors (SSRIs):

    a) have more side effects
    b) are more dangerous in terms of overdose
    c) are less expensive
    d) were not discovered accidentally

MC/Mod
Pg:187
kind:c
Ans:(d)

5.77: Prozac (fluoxetine) is:

    a) an SSRI
    b) the same as imipramine
    c) an MAO inhibitor
    d) a tricyclic

MC/Mod
Pg:188
kind:f
Ans:(a)

5.78: An antidepressant medication which is prescribed more than twice as often as the next most commonly prescribed antidepressant is:

    a) Prozac   b) imipramine
    c) lithium   d) Valium

MC/Easy
Pg:188
kind:f
Ans:(a)

5.79: Prozac is by far the most widely used antidepressant drug. The popularity of Prozac can be attributed largely to its:

    a) low cost
    b) additional use as a weight-loss tool
    c) minimal side effects
    d) over-the-counter availability

MC/Mod
Pg:188
kind:c
Ans:(c)

5.80: The most difficult issue in the evaluation of the effects of light treatment for seasonal affective disorder (SAD) has been:

    a) controlling for radiation
    b) finding the right spectrum of light
    c) controlling for placebo effects
    d) the long latency period before treatment is effective

MC/Mod
Pg:189
kind:c
Ans:(c)

True-False Questions

5.81: Mood refers to a pattern of observable behaviors such as crying, yelling, and smiling.

TF/Mod
Pg:152
kind:c
Ans:False

5.82: Clinical depression is defined by emotional symptoms, not cognitive or behavioral symptoms.

TF/Mod
Pg:152
kind:c
Ans:False

5.83: A person who has had one episode of mania would be diagnosed with a bipolar disorder.

TF/Diff
Pg:153
kind:a
Ans:True

5.84: There is no clearcut line dividing normal sadness from a depressed mood associated with clinical depression.

TF/Mod
Pg:155
kind:c
Ans:True

5.85: Anxiety commonly co-occurs with depression.

TF/Easy
Pg:159
kind:f
Ans:True

5.86: An early name for manic depression was dementia praecox.

TF/Mod
Pg:160
kind:f
Ans:False

5.87: Most people with unipolar mood disorder experience a single, isolated episode of major depression without repeated episodes.

TF/Mod
Pg:161
kind:c
Ans:False

5.88: Manic episodes are involved in Bipolar II disorder.

TF/Mod
Pg:161
kind:f
Ans:False

5.89: Postpartum onset of depression or mania refers to onset of problems in a mother soon after childbirth.

TF/Easy
Pg:163
kind:f
Ans:True

5.90: Most evidence points to clearcut differences between unipolar and bipolar disorders in terms of age of onset and in terms of prognosis.

TF/Mod
Pg:164
kind:c
Ans:True

5.91: Bipolar mood disorder is more common in women than in men.

TF/Mod
Pg:166
kind:f
Ans:False

5.92: Clinical depression is a phenomenon primarily limited to Western and urban societies.

TF/Mod
Pg:167
kind:f
Ans:False

5.93: Rates of clinical depression are especially high among the elderly.

TF/Diff
Pg:168
kind:f
Ans:False

5.94: Rates of completed suicide are higher among females.

TF/Mod
Pg:169
kind:f
Ans:False

5.95: Brown and Harris' (1978) study of stress and depression in women found that unipolar depression was most often associated with an accumulation of ordinary hassles and difficulties rather than any one single stressful life event.

TF/Mod
Pg:171
kind:c
Ans:False

5.96: Beck views a depressed person's critical self-statements as a reflection of anger toward others.

TF/Easy
Pg:174
kind:c
Ans:False

5.97: Research on cognitive distortions shows that, compared to nondepressed people, depressed people show more cognitive distortions primarily while they are depressed, not beforehand.

TF/Mod
Pg:174
kind:c
Ans:True

5.98: The schemas most clearly related to depression are those associated with self-evaluation and relationships.

TF/Mod
Pg:174
kind:c
Ans:True

5.99: According to Beck's model of depression, cognitive distortions are the sole cause of depression.

TF/Mod
Pg:174
kind:c
Ans:False

5.100: Abramson, Alloy, and colleagues view a "depressogenic" attributional style as one characterized by a tendency to explain negative events in terms of internal, stable, and global factors.

TF/Mod
Pg:174
kind:c
Ans:True

5.101: A depressogenic attributional style is thought to be a sufficient cause of depression.

TF/Mod
Pg:175
kind:c
Ans:False

5.102: According to the learning model of depression, a depressed person's behavior may be initially unintentionally reinforced by friends' attempts to provide comfort and support.

TF/Mod
Pg:176
kind:c
Ans:True

99

5.103: Research shows that the maladaptive relationship patterns shown by depressed persons are only evident during the episode of depression, not before or after.

TF/Mod
Pg:176
kind:c
Ans:False

5.104: Among the relatives of patients with bipolar mood disorder, the risk for both bipolar and unipolar disorder is much higher than in the general population.

TF/Diff
Pg:178
kind:f
Ans:True

5.105: MAO inhibitors work by blocking the breakdown of serotonin and norepinephrine.

TF/Diff
Pg:180
kind:c
Ans:True

5.106: The catecholamine hypothesis of depression held that depression was associated with higher levels of norepinephrine.

TF/Diff
Pg:181
kind:c
Ans:False

5.107: In the dexamethasone suppression test (DST), synthetic hormone is introduced into the body. Nondepressed persons usually respond to this test by producing less of the natural hormone cortisol.

TF/Diff
Pg:182
kind:c
Ans:True

5.108: The primary disadvantage of analogue studies is the questionable generalizability to situations outside the laboratory.

TF/Mod
Pg:183
kind:c
Ans:True

5.109: Electroconvulsive therapy (ECT) is more effective for the treatment of schizophrenia than depression.

TF/Easy
Pg:186
kind:f
Ans:False

5.110: Electroconvulsive therapy (ECT) is typically administered two or three times a week for several weeks.

TF/Mod
Pg:186
kind:f
Ans:True

5.111: Tricyclics block the reuptake of serotonin specifically, not other neurotransmitters.

TF/Diff
Pg:187
kind:f
Ans:False

5.112: Lithium carbonate is more often used to treat
bipolar disorder than to treat unipolar disorder.

TF/Mod
Pg:188
kind:f
Ans:True

Essay Questions

5.113: What are the two primary issues central to the debate about
definitions of mood disorders?

Answer: (1) to use broad definitions or narrow ones; e.g., whether to
include regular unhappiness and grief under the category of
depression. (2) the issue of heterogeneity; i.e., are the various
mood disorders different forms of one disorder, or different
disorders?

ES Moderate Page: 160 kind: c

5.114: Research consistently finds lower rates of depression among the
elderly than among other age groups. However, it is possible that
this finding is due to how the research was conducted, not actual
differences in the rate of depression across age groups. What are
some of the methodological factors that might explain the lower
rate of depression found among the elderly?

Answer: (1) some of the elderly population has already died at the time of
data collection, and it is possible that some of the deceased
would have been counted as depressed before they died; (2) elderly
people grew up before World War II, and rates of depression
increased in our society after World War II; (3) depression may be
mistaken for senility in the elderly.

ES Moderate Page: 168 kind: c

5.115: Discuss methodological problems that are involved in studying the association between stressors and depression. How have these issues been addressed in research suggesting an association between stress and depression?

Answer: (1) Retrospective reports can be biased by a negative world view. Also, depression could lead to a stressful event (such as being fired), rather than vice versa. (2) Researchers have addressed these problems by getting detailed information about the stressor and its context, in order to obtain objective ratings of whether the event would be considered stressful; they have counted as stressful only "fateful" events that cannot be the consequence of depression; and they have used prospective designs to analyze the temporal sequence of stressors and depression.

ES Difficult Pages: 170-171 kind: c

5.116: Describe the research results suggesting that there is a greater genetic influence on bipolar disorder than on unipolar disorder.

Answer: (1) There is a greater difference in the concordance rates for MZ and DZ twins in the case of bipolar disorder than in the case of unipolar disorder. (2) The rate of bipolar disorder in family members of unipolar patients is similar to the rate in the general population, but the rate of unipolar disorder in family members of bipolar patients is higher than the rate in the general population.

ES Moderate Page: 178 kind: c

5.117: Discuss the two major limitations of genetic linkage studies.

Answer: (1) The gene(s) responsible for a trait may be different depending on the pedigree. This is the issue of genetic heterogeneity. (2) It is not possible to establish a link unless a single gene of main effect is responsible for the trait or disorder. In some traits or disorders, multiple genes are responsible.

ES Moderate Page: 180 kind: c

5.118: Research on the animal model of depression is sometimes used as an example of how environmental and biological factors interact to produce depression. Describe the research results which indicate that the association between stress (uncontrollable shock) and "depressed" behavior in rats may be mediated by biological processes.

Answer: Antidepressant medications reverse or prevent the behavioral effects of uncontrollable shock in rats. Also, uncontrollable shocks cause a drop in the level of norepinephrine in the brain; only rats who show this drop in norepinephrine in response to stress then become depressed.

ES Difficult Page: 182 kind: c

Chapter 6
Anxiety Disorders

Multiple Choice Questions

6.1: Agoraphobia refers to an exaggerated fear of:

    a) water
    b) situations where escape is difficult
    c) insects
    d) high places

MC/Mod
Pg:194
kind:f
Ans:(b)

6.2: Which situation would an agoraphobic be most likely to avoid or fear?

    a) sitting in the middle of a row in a crowded theater
    b) being at the top of a tall building
    c) touching an insect
    d) swimming in a backyard pool

MC/Mod
Pg:194
kind:a
Ans:(a)

6.3: An agoraphobic may feel terrified of crowds because:

    a) she fears people
    b) she is paranoid
    c) she has low self-esteem
    d) she fears not being able to escape

MC/Mod
Pg:196
kind:c
Ans:(d)

6.4: Anxiety is a reaction to:

    a) an immediate threat from the environment
    b) avoidance
    c) impaired insight
    d) anticipated future negative events

MC/Mod
Pg:198
kind:c
Ans:(d)

6.5: In contrast to anxiety, fear:

    a) is more general
    b) is out of proportion to threats from the environment
    c) is associated with anticipation of future problems
    d) occurs in the face of immediate danger

MC/Mod
Pg:198
kind:c
Ans:(d)

6.6: In contrast to fear, anxiety:

MC/Mod
Pg:198
kind:c
Ans:(d)

a) is more specific
b) occurs in the face of immediate danger
c) helps organize behavioral responses to real threats
d) is out of proportion to threats from the environment

6.7: Which of the following is typically associated with anxious mood?

MC/Mod
Pg:199
kind:c
Ans:(a)

a) pessimism and negative self-evaluation
b) organization and rehearsal of adaptive responses
c) preoccupation with other people
d) poor insight into the worry

6.8: According to Barlow, anxious apprehension involves which of the following?

MC/Diff
Pg:199
kind:c
Ans:(b)

a) specific negative emotions
b) sense of uncontrollability
c) preoccupation with others
d) immediate danger

6.9: Worry is a relatively uncontrollable sequence of negative emotional thoughts and images concerned with:

MC/Mod
Pg:199
kind:c
Ans:(c)

a) immediate danger
b) physiological hyperarousal
c) possible future threats or future dangers
d) absence of positive affect

6.10: According to Borkovec's research, most worriers are preoccupied with:

MC/Mod
Pg:199
kind:f
Ans:(c)

a) visual images
b) bodily or somatic complaints
c) self-talk and verbal material
d) immediate dangers or threats

6.11: In contrast to normal worrying, pathological worrying:

    a) focuses on possible future events
    b) involves a feeling that the worry can't be controlled
    c) focuses on immediate dangers
    d) is associated with both positive and negative affect

MC/Mod
Pg:199
kind:c
Ans:(b)

6.12: Compared to anxiety, a panic attack:

    a) is less like a normal fear response
    b) has a less sudden onset
    c) is less intense
    d) is more focused

MC/Mod
Pg:199
kind:c
Ans:(d)

6.13: Panic is like a normal fear response, but it:

    a) is triggered at an inappropriate time
    b) has a slower onset
    c) is less intense
    d) involves less anxiety

MC/Mod
Pg:199
kind:c
Ans:(a)

6.14: According to DSM-IV, a panic attack must:

    a) show gradual buildup over several days
    b) reach a peak within 10 minutes
    c) involve a blend of several negative emotions
    d) involve preoccupation with words rather than images

MC/Mod
Pg:200
kind:f
Ans:(b)

6.15: Panic attacks that occur only in specific, predictable circumstances are considered to be:

    a) anxious apprehension
    b) phobias
    c) natural fear responses
    d) situationally cued

MC/Easy
Pg:200
kind:c
Ans:(d)

6.16: A panic attack is said to be "situationally cued" if it:

    a) occurs without warning or "out of the blue"
    b) is triggered by a real, not imagined, danger
    c) only occurs in predictable situations
    d) is triggered by an imagined, not real, danger

MC/Mod
Pg:200
kind:c
Ans:(c)

6.17: Compared to panic attacks, phobias:

    a) are less narrowly defined
    b) are more narrowly defined
    c) involve more physiological reactions
    d) involve more worrying

MC/Mod
Pg:200
kind:c
Ans:(b)

6.18: In contrast to a fear, a phobia involves:

    a) more self-preoccupation
    b) a more general focus
    c) attempts to avoid an object
    d) less intense physiological responses

MC/Mod
Pg:200
kind:c
Ans:(c)

6.19: Approximately what percentage of normal people experience obsessions in one form or another?

    a) 1%   b) 10%
    c) 50%   d) 90%

MC/Easy
Pg:202
kind:f
Ans:(d)

6.20: Clinical obsessions differ from normal obsessions:

    a) in that they are more visually oriented
    b) in that they are more likely to be acted upon
    c) in degree rather than kind
    d) in the content of the images

MC/Diff
Pg:202
kind:c
Ans:(c)

6.21: Compulsions are:

    a) intrusive, unwanted thoughts
    b) a type of obsession
    c) irrational, repetitive behaviors
    d) normal feelings of drive or ambition

MC/Mod
Pg:202
kind:f
Ans:(c)

6.22: Compulsions:

    a) reduce anxiety, don't increase pleasure
    b) reduce anxiety, increase pleasure
    c) increase anxiety, increase pleasure
    d) increase anxiety, don't increase pleasure

MC/Diff
Pg:202
kind:c
Ans:(a)

6.23: The 2 most common forms of compulsion involve:

    a) counting and collecting
    b) eating and dressing
    c) escape and avoidance
    d) checking and cleaning

MC/Easy
Pg:202
kind:f
Ans:(d)

6.24: A common complication associated with anxiety disorders is:

    a) psychosis
    b) personality disorder
    c) substance abuse
    d) mania

MC/Easy
Pg:203
kind:f
Ans:(c)

6.25: According to Clark and Watson's model of negative emotional responses, one distinction between anxiety and depression is that:

    a) general distress is specific to anxiety
    b) negative affect is specific to anxiety
    c) physiological hyperarousal is specific to anxiety
    d) absence of positive affect is specific to anxiety

MC/Mod
Pg:204
kind:c
Ans:(c)

6.26: According to Clark and Watson, one thing that anxiety and depression have in common is:

    a) physiological hyperarousal
    b) general distress and high negative affect
    c) absence of positive affect
    d) absence of negative affect

MC/Mod
Pg:204
kind:c
Ans:(b)

6.27: Anxiety disorders did not play a prominent role in psychiatric classification systems in the 1800s, probably because:

    a) there were many fewer cases then
    b) they were seen as a physiological, not psychological, problem
    c) very few cases were treated in institutions where they would be seen by psychiatrists
    d) they were seen as a moral or religious problem

MC/Diff
Pg:205
kind:c
Ans:(c)

6.28: "Psychasthenia" was a term coined by:

MC/Easy
Pg:205
kind:f
Ans:(b)

a) Barlow   b) Janet
c) Freud   d) Klein

6.29: "Psychasthenia" refers to:

MC/Diff
Pg:205
kind:c
Ans:(d)

a) a feeling of numbness during a panic attack
b) hysterical neurosis
c) induced hypnosis, used to treat phobia
d) many different symptoms associated with
   anxiety, including indecisiveness and rigidity

6.30: Janet's description of the early stages of
      psychasthenia bears a close resemblance to current
      conceptualizations of:

MC/Mod
Pg:205
kind:c
Ans:(d)

a) generalized anxiety disorder
b) phobia
c) panic attack
d) obsessive compulsive disorder

6.31: In DSM-I and DSM-II, anxiety disorders were grouped
      under the general heading of:

MC/Mod
Pg:205
kind:f
Ans:(c)

a) personality disorders
b) psychasthenia
c) neuroses
d) mood disorders

6.32: In the past, hysterical neuroses were grouped with
      other anxiety disorders under "neuroses." Now they
      are categorized as:

MC/Mod
Pg:206
kind:f
Ans:(a)

a) somatoform and dissociative disorders
b) psychosomatic illnesses
c) personality disorders
d) mood disorders

6.33: European psychiatry tends to see the various
      symptoms of anxiety as:

MC/Diff
Pg:206
kind:c
Ans:(d)

a) specific types of disorder, each with its own
   etiology
b) more physiological than psychological
c) subtypes of psychasthenia
d) a generalized condition

6.34: One of the key changes in the DSM-III   MC/Diff
       subclassification descriptions of anxiety disorders   Pg:206
       was based on the idea that: kind:c
                                                                   Ans:(d)

       a) some anxiety is neurotic, some isn't
       b) patients with panic disorder don't respond to
          medication
       c) some patients with generalized anxiety disorder
          also show phobias
       d) some people with panic attacks develop
          agoraphobia, others don't

6.35: The DSM-I and DSM-II category of "free-floating   MC/Diff
       anxiety" was made into 2 categories in the DSM-III.   Pg:206
       These 2 new categories were: kind:c
                                                                   Ans:(d)

       a) psychasthenia and obsessive-compulsive disorder
       b) anxiety disorder and neurosis
       c) somatoform and dissociative disorder
       d) generalized anxiety disorder and panic disorder

6.36: In DSM-IV, panic disorders are subdivided based on   MC/Mod
       the presence or absence of: Pg:206
                                                                   kind:c
       a) personality disorder   Ans:(b)
       b) agoraphobia
       c) posttraumatic stress disorder
       d) obsessions

6.37: Social phobia is most similar to: MC/Mod
                                                                   Pg:207
       a) specific phobia   kind:c
       b) agoraphobia   Ans:(a)
       c) panic disorder
       d) generalized anxiety disorder

6.38: In order to be diagnosed with obsessive-compulsive   MC/Mod
       disorder, the person must: Pg:208
                                                                   kind:f
       a) show both obsessions and compulsions   Ans:(c)
       b) show free-floating anxiety
       c) realize that the obsessions or compulsions are
          unreasonable
       d) have a history of phobias

6.39: Barney has many overdue bills that he cannot pay. He finds himself constantly thinking about them at work, as he tries to sleep, and when he exercises. According to DSM-IV, Barney's experience would not be classified as an obsession or as generalized anxiety disorder because:

MC/Mod
Pg:208
kind:a
Ans:(a)

   a) the thoughts are about a real problem
   b) he is still able to function at work and at home
   c) it would be classified as a compulsion
   d) he does not feel compelled to do anything about the problem

6.40: An essential element of the diagnosis of obsessive compulsive disorder is that:

MC/Mod
Pg:208
kind:f
Ans:(a)

   a) the person tries to suppress or neutralize the unwanted thoughts
   b) the person makes no attempt to ignore the unwanted thoughts
   c) the obsessions develop in response to the compulsions
   d) the person engages in compulsions, which increase anxiety

6.41: Approximately what percentage of persons who would qualify for a diagnosis of some type of anxiety disorder present themselves for treatment?

MC/Mod
Pg:208
kind:f
Ans:(a)

   a) 5%   b) 25%
   c) 75%   d) 95%

6.42: The most common form of anxiety disorder is:

MC/Easy
Pg:208
kind:f
Ans:(a)

   a) phobia
   b) generalized anxiety disorder
   c) panic attacks
   d) post traumatic stress disorder

6.43: Rates of anxiety disorder found by the Epidemiologic Catchment Area (ECA) study may be inflated because:

MC/Diff
Pg:209
kind:c
Ans:(c)

a) they included cases of mixed anxiety-depression disorder
b) they included cases of hysterical neurosis
c) they may have been based on excessively broad definitions
d) anxiety disorders are more common in the U.S. than Canada

6.44: In nonwestern societies, anxiety may be most frequently associated with family or religious concerns. In western societies, anxiety may be most frequently associated with:

MC/Diff
Pg:210
Ans:(b)

a) personal appearance
b) work
c) intimate relationships
d) financial concerns

6.45: Which anxiety disorder is equally common in men and women?

MC/Mod
Pg:210
kind:f
Ans:(b)

a) specific phobia   b) social phobia
c) agoraphobia   d) panic disorder

6.46: Cross-cultural studies of panic disorder show that one symptom that appears to be universal is:

MC/Mod
Pg:210
kind:f
Ans:(d)

a) fear of dying
b) choking or smothering sensations
c) phobic avoidance
d) heart palpitations

6.47: Freud's view of the adaptive function of anxiety was that:

MC/Diff
Pg:211
kind:c
Ans:(d)

a) repression leads to anxiety
b) anxiety is due to incomplete repression
c) anxiety causes people to act out aggressive and sexual impulses
d) signal anxiety leads to repression

6.48: According to attachment theory, anxiety is:

    a) a learned response to neglect
    b) a defense against sexual impulses
    c) an innate response to separation from the
       caregiver
    d) associated with threatening memories

MC/Mod
Pg:212
kind:c
Ans:(c)

6.49: The "strange situation" is:

    a) an outdated term for events eliciting social
       phobias
    b) a treatment exercise for agoraphobics
    c) a Freudian term for confusion when recalling
       childhood trauma
    d) a research procedure for studying attachment

MC/Mod
Pg:212
kind:f
Ans:(d)

6.50: Which describes securely attached infants?

    a) keep playing calmly when mother returns after
       absence
    b) show irritation when mother returns after
       absence
    c) do not cry when mother leaves
    d) cry when mother leaves

MC/Diff
Pg:212
kind:c
Ans:(d)

6.51: A child cries a lot when the mother leaves the
room. When the mother returns, the child cries for
another 10 minutes, seemingly unable to be
consoled. Which of the following attachment styles
best describes this relationship?

    a) secure
    b) avoidant
    c) ambivalent/resistant
    d) disorganized

MC/Diff
Pg:212
kind:a
Ans:(c)

6.52: Harriet is in a car accident. She then becomes
fearful of riding in cars. The car accident is:

    a) a source of signal anxiety
    b) the conditioning event
    c) a symbol of loss
    d) important if it is also associated with
       interpersonal conflict

MC/Diff
Pg:213
kind:a
Ans:(b)

6.53: You're walking along, and a car drives by and honks   MC/Diff
right next to you. Your heart starts pounding and   Pg:213
you're startled. A few minutes later another car   kind:a
comes by and you feel a little on edge and nervous.   Ans:(c)
In this scenario, the horn honking is the:

a) conditioned stimulus
b) conditioned response
c) unconditioned stimulus
d) unconditioned response

6.54: Barbara has been afraid of cats ever since one   MC/Diff
brushed against her leg just as she witnessed a   Pg:214
terrible train wreck. If this scenario were to be   kind:a
viewed in classical conditioning terms, what is the   Ans:(b)
conditioned response?

a) fear experienced at the sight of the train
wreck
b) fear of cats
c) the cat brushing against her leg
d) the noise of the train wreck

6.55: Seligman proposed revisions of classical   MC/Diff
conditioning models of phobias in part based on   Pg:214
evidence that: kind:c
    Ans:(a)

a) phobic responses seem to develop only in
response to certain stimuli
b) phobic responses are easy to extinguish in the
laboratory
c) laboratory studies can often induce fear
responses after only 1 trial
d) conditioned fear responses learned in the
laboratory are difficult to extinguish

6.56: Seligman's preparedness theory of phobic   MC/Mod
acquisition holds that phobias develop in response   Pg:214
to: kind:c
    Ans:(a)

a) objects and situations that humans are
biologically "wired" to fear
b) any neutral stimulus paired with an
unconditioned stimulus
c) objects with symbolic associations to sex and
aggression
d) novel things to which the person has had little
exposure

114

6.57: Rhesus monkeys that have been reared in a   MC/Diff
       laboratory show little fear of snakes until they   Pg:215
       watch other monkeys who show fear of snakes. This   kind:c
       is evidence for: Ans:(c)

       a) unconditioned responses becoming conditioned
       b) conditioned stimuli becoming unconditioned
       c) vicarious learning
       d) a primacy effect

6.58: Many children in London during World War II   MC/Mod
       experienced bombing raids while they were staying   Pg:215
       in underground shelters, but very few developed any   kind:c
       irrational phobic responses to things associated   Ans:(d)
       with the shelters, such as tunnels or the dark.
       Anecdotal evidence suggests that this was because:

       a) the children knew they were safe inside
       b) the children were usually prepared for the
          bombing
       c) the children knew the war was for a good cause
       d) the adults around the children appeared calm

6.59: Dogs in a laboratory are required to discriminate   MC/Diff
       between 2 virtually identical geometric figures.   Pg:216
       The dogs show behaviors similar to neurotic human   kind:c
       behaviors, such as agitation and an increased   Ans:(b)
       startle response. Psychologists believe that this
       is because:

       a) the visual strain exhausts the dogs
       b) the task is unpredictable and uncontrollable
       c) the dogs' agitation is actually normal
          excitement about novelty
       d) the dogs' agitation is due to being confined,
          not due to the task

115

6.60: According to the idea of "catastrophic misinterpretation," an important cognitive element in the development of panic disorder is exemplified by:

MC/Mod
Pg:216
kind:c
Ans:(c)

a) a belief that you are the only one with panic disorder
b) a belief that you should be able to control the panic attacks
c) interpreting rapid heart beats as a heart attack
d) poor insight to associated interpersonal difficulties

6.61: Experimental subjects, all diagnosed with panic disorder, were administered carbon-dioxide-enriched air. Some subjects believed that they could control the amount of carbon dioxide; others believed they could not control it. Which result occurred?

MC/Mod
Pg:218
kind:f
Ans:(c)

a) rates of panic depended only on the amount of carbon dioxide
b) rates of panic depended only on the amount of perceived control
c) panic increased among those who believed they had no control
d) panic increased among those who believed they had control

6.62: According to Borkovec, worrying is a primarily verbal-linguistic event that serves the function of avoiding unpleasant somatic activation through:

MC/Diff
Pg:219
kind:c
Ans:(c)

a) rehearsal of coping strategies
b) repetition of "what if?" questions
c) suppression of imagery
d) focus on the future, not the present

6.63: According to cognitive models of anxiety (such as Borkovec's model), worrying is unproductive because it distracts a person from focusing on:

MC/Mod
Pg:219
kind:c
Ans:(b)

a) self-evaluation
b) active coping behaviors
c) images
d) suppression

6.64: Thought suppression is:

    a) an active attempt to stop thinking about something
    b) an unconscious process that keeps memories from awareness
    c) usually the result of trauma
    d) an attention deficit caused by intrusive images

MC/Mod
Pg:219
kind:f
Ans:(a)

6.65: According to Wegner, trying to rid your mind of a distressing or unwanted thought:

    a) will help relax you and take away physiological cues
    b) might actually make the thought more intrusive
    c) is a necessary first step in eliminating anxiety disorder
    d) is most easily accomplished when physiologically aroused

MC/Mod
Pg:219
kind:c
Ans:(b)

6.66: The episodic nature of obsessive compulsive disorder symptoms is thought to be related to:

    a) unwanted thoughts disappearing in association with strong emotions
    b) unwanted thoughts reappearing in association with strong emotions
    c) cycles of activity in neurotransmitters
    d) cycles of activity in lactate concentrations

MC/Diff
Pg:219
kind:c
Ans:(b)

6.67: One important element in the development of social phobias may be a biologically-based preparedness to fear:

    a) persons in positions of power
    b) large crowds
    c) faces that appear angry or critical
    d) unrelated persons more than biologically related persons

MC/Mod
Pg:220
kind:c
Ans:(c)

6.68: In which situation might a person show a social phobia?　　　　MC/Mod Pg:220 kind:a Ans:(b)

   a) standing in a large crowd at a concert
   b) performing at a concert
   c) feeling sexually attracted to the performer at a concert
   d) having one's name called over the loudspeaker at a concert

6.69: Early studies lumping all anxiety disorders together found that compared to relatives of controls, first degree relatives of anxiety patients showed rates of anxiety that were:　　MC/Mod Pg:220 kind:f Ans:(b)

   a) 5 times as high　　　b) 2 times as high
   c) equally as high　　　d) half as high

6.70: Studies of the genetics of panic disorder and generalized anxiety disorder show that first degree relatives of patients with panic disorder show:　　MC/Diff Pg:220 kind:f Ans:(d)

   a) average rates of panic, average rates of GAD
   b) average rates of panic, higher rates of GAD
   c) higher than average rates of panic and GAD
   d) higher than average rates of panic, not GAD

6.71: Family members of obsessive-compulsive disorder (OCD) patients show:　　MC/Diff Pg:221 kind:f Ans:(d)

   a) lower rates of OCD
   b) lower rates of anxiety disorders other than OCD
   c) higher rates of OCD
   d) higher rates of anxiety disorders other than OCD

6.72: Genetic studies of inheritance suggest validity for which type of classification with regard to obsessive compulsive disorder (OCD), generalized anxiety disorder (GAD), panic disorder, and other anxiety disorders?　　MC/Diff Pg:221 kind:c Ans:(a)

   a) GAD distinct from panic disorder
   b) OCD distinct from GAD
   c) GAD lumped in with other anxiety disorders
   d) panic disorder lumped in with other anxiety disorders

118

6.73: A research technique for inducing panic attack in patients with panic disorder is:

a) infusion of lactate (lactic acid)
b) administration of clomipramine
c) reducing carbon dioxide
d) MAO inhibition

MC/Mod
Pg:222
kind:c
Ans:(a)

6.74: The infusion of lactate can:

a) decrease panic symptoms in patients with panic disorder
b) decrease panic symptoms in normals
c) induce a panic attack in patients with panic disorder
d) induce a panic attack in normals

MC/Mod
Pg:223
kind:f
Ans:(c)

6.75: Positron emission tomography (PET) scans of panic disorder patients who have just had a panic attack after being infused with lactate show increased blood flow to which area of the brain?

a) frontal lobe   b) temporal lobe
c) occipital lobe   d) corpus callosum

MC/Mod
Pg:223
kind:f
Ans:(b)

6.76: Studies of the use of imipramine (Tofranil) with agoraphobics show:

a) increased anticipatory anxiety, but not panic
b) increased anxiety, but not anticipatory anxiety
c) reduced anticipatory anxiety, but not panic
d) reduced panic attacks, but not anticipatory anxiety

MC/Mod
Pg:223
kind:c
Ans:(d)

6.77: According to Klein, agoraphobic reactions may be triggered by a misfiring of biological signals associated with:

a) migraine   b) suffocation
c) starvation   d) depression

MC/Mod
Pg:223
kind:c
Ans:(b)

6.78: Klein views the essential symptom of panic as:

a) shortness of breath   b) heart palpitations
c) sweatiness   d) upset stomach

MC/Mod
Pg:223
kind:f
Ans:(a)

6.79: Desensitization involves:

    a) dampening of physiological reactions with
       medication
    b) insight to unconscious motivations
    c) gradual exposure to feared objects while
       relaxed
    d) suppression of phobic thoughts

MC/Mod
Pg:225
kind:f
Ans:(c)

6.80: Flooding refers to:

    a) the recovery of repressed memories
    b) exposure to highly feared objects
    c) the rebound effect after thought suppression
    d) the side effects of anti-anxiety medications

MC/Mod
Pg:225
kind:f
Ans:(b)

6.81: Effective behavioral treatment of obsessive
compulsive disorder combines exposure to the
anxiety-provoking situation with:

    a) encouragement to use compulsive behaviors to
       reduce anxiety
    b) discussion of unconscious motivations
    c) prevention of the compulsive behaviors
    d) thought suppression

MC/Mod
Pg:226
kind:c
Ans:(c)

6.82: Exposure and response prevention is most effective
in the treatment of:

    a) pure obsessions
    b) compulsive rituals
    c) thought suppression
    d) more severe cases of obsessive compulsive
       disorder

MC/Mod
Pg:226
kind:f
Ans:(b)

6.83: A cognitive therapist asks a patient to say what he
assumes would happen if his worst case scenario
actually happened. The patient says, "If I fail
this test, I'll never get into graduate school."
The next step in decatastrophisizing would be to
help the patient:

    a) imagine not getting into graduate school,
       paired with relaxation
    b) recognize the gross exaggeration of this idea
    c) use more effective all-or-none thinking
    d) use thought suppression to ignore such thoughts

MC/Mod
Pg:228
kind:a
Ans:(b)

6.84: Benzodiazepines are: MC/Mod
                                                          Pg:228
    a) antidepressants   kind:f
    b) receptor sites of GABA   Ans:(d)
    c) antipsychotics
    d) minor tranquilizers

6.85: Benzodiazepines: MC/Mod
                                                          Pg:228
    a) inhibit activity of GABA   kind:c
    b) increase activity of GABA   Ans:(a)
    c) are a form of tricyclic
    d) are a form of MAO inhibitors

6.86: Benzodiazepines are most effective for treating: MC/Mod
                                                          Pg:228
    a) phobias   kind:f
    b) obsessive compulsive disorder   Ans:(c)
    c) generalized anxiety disorder
    d) rumination

6.87: The most serious adverse side effect of   MC/Mod
      benzodiazepines is that they: Pg:229
                                                          kind:f
    a) are potentially addictive   Ans:(a)
    b) interfere with motor skills
    c) can cause weight loss, leading to chemical
       imbalance
    d) can cause organ damage

6.88: For treatment of panic disorder, many psychiatrists MC/Mod
      prefer: Pg:229
                                                          kind:f
    a) benzodiazepines, because they are not addictive   Ans:(b)
    b) tricyclics, because they are not addictive
    c) benzodiazepines, because they have few side
       effects
    d) tricyclics, because they have few side effects

True-False Questions

6.89: Many patients who are anxious are also depressed.   TF/Mod
                                                          Pg:194
                                                          kind:f
                                                          Ans:True

6.90: Persons with anxiety disorders usually show poor insight into their condition.

TF/Mod
Pg:198
kind:f
Ans:False

6.91: At low levels, anxiety can be adaptive because it serves as a signal that the person must prepare for an upcoming event.

TF/Mod
Pg:198
kind:c
Ans:True

6.92: Panic attacks are usually defined in terms of somatic or physiological sensations.

TF/Easy
Pg:199
kind:f
Ans:True

6.93: Fear of heights is known as acrophobia.

TF/Mod
Pg:201
kind:f
Ans:True

6.94: Obsessions are characterized by unwanted, intrusive thoughts.

TF/Mod
Pg:202
kind:c
Ans:True

6.95: Gambling and drug use are not considered true compulsions because they are pleasurable activities.

TF/Mod
Pg:202
kind:f
Ans:True

6.96: Compulsive behaviors are completely automatic and are associated with a complete loss of voluntary control.

TF/Mod
Pg:202
kind:c
Ans:False

6.97: Phobias, panic, and obsessions are all characterized as anxiety disorders, but there is little overlap between their features.

TF/Mod
Pg:203
kind:c
Ans:False

6.98: Very few people meet the criteria for more than one anxiety disorder at a time.

TF/Easy
Pg:203
kind:f
Ans:False

6.99: Freud believed that the underlying causes of various anxiety disorders were different, depending on the specific type of disorder.

TF/Diff
Pg:205
kind:c
Ans:False

6.100: In the DSM-III, the concept of neurosis was dropped as a general organizing principle.

TF/Diff
Pg:206
kind:f
Ans:True

6.101: A person with a social phobia is afraid of other people.

TF/Mod
Pg:207
kind:f
Ans:False

6.102: According to the Epidemiologic Catchment Area study, the various forms of anxiety disorder (phobia, obsession, compulsion, extreme worry) represent the most common form of abnormal behavior in the U.S.

TF/Mod
Pg:208
kind:f
Ans:True

6.103: To be diagnosed with obsessive-compulsive disorder, a person must show both obsessions and related compulsions.

TF/Mod
Pg:208
kind:f
Ans:False

6.104: Estimates of the frequency of anxiety disorders are usually based on community samples because most people with anxiety disorders do not seek treatment.

TF/Diff
Pg:208
kind:f
Ans:True

6.105: The Epidemiologic Catchment Area study found that anxiety disorders are more common than any other form of mental disorder.

TF/Mod
Pg:208
kind:f
Ans:True

6.106: Anxiety disorders are generally more common among females than males.

TF/Mod
Pg:209
kind:f
Ans:True

6.107: The primary defense mechanism thought to be at work in obsessive-compulsive disorder is reaction formation.

TF/Mod
Pg:211
kind:c
Ans:True

6.108: The anxiety disorder that is most closely linked to interpersonal conflicts is agoraphobia.

TF/Diff
Pg:213
kind:c
Ans:True

6.109: Stressful experiences involving loss appear to be more associated with depression than with anxiety.

TF/Mod
Pg:214
kind:c
Ans:True

6.110: Rhesus monkeys that have been reared in a laboratory with no exposure to monkeys reared in the wild show little fear of a toy snake.

TF/Mod
Pg:215
kind:f
Ans:True

6.111: Compared to specific phobias, social phobias are more likely to develop through vicarious learning.

TF/Diff
Pg:216
kind:c
Ans:False

6.112: Worry is generally conceptualized as an emotional, not cognitive, state.

TF/Mod
Pg:217
kind:c
Ans:False

6.113: One way that obsessive-compulsive disorder (OCD) patients differ from normals with obsessive thoughts is that OCD patients try more vigorously to resist the thoughts.

TF/Diff
Pg:219
kind:c
Ans:True

6.114: Obsessive-compulsive disorder appears to run in families.

TF/Mod
Pg:221
kind:f
Ans:False

6.115: Overall, genetic factors do not seem to play a large role in the etiology of anxiety disorders.

TF/Mod
Pg:221
kind:f
Ans:False

6.116: According to Donald Klein's hypothesis, panic is associated with the overactivation of the same biological pathways as those associated with fear.

TF/Diff
Pg:223
kind:c
Ans:False

6.117: A statistically significant result is not necessarily clinically important.

TF/Mod
Pg:227
kind:c
Ans:True

6.118: Benzodiazepines are more addictive than tricyclics.

TF/Mod
Pg:229
kind:f
Ans:True

Essay Questions

6.119: Define phobia. Describe the difference between a phobia and normal fear. Given an example of the difference between a phobia and normal fear.

Answer: (1) A phobia is the expression of an immediate, exaggerated, sometimes irrational fear reaction when in the proximity of an object that is not really dangerous, and/or avoidance of the object, which interferes with daily life. (2) In contrast to normal fear, phobia involves attempts to avoid an object that others do not find dangerous. (3) A person who fears cats may prefer not to be around them, and may show physiological arousal when close to a cat; a person who is phobic of cats would have an immediate fear reaction upon seeing a cat, and the person's attempts to avoid getting closer to the cat might interfere with whatever the person was doing at the time.

ES   Moderate   Page: 200   kind: c

6.120: Describe the relationship between obsessions and compulsions in obsessive-compulsive disorder. Do both have to be present for the diagnosis of OCD to be made? Which typically comes first? What is their functional relationship?

Answer: Most patients with OCD show both obsessions and compulsions, but this is not necessary for the diagnosis. Compulsions develop to neutralize the obsessions and related anxiety (which typically come first).

ES   Moderate   Page: 207   kind: c

125

6.121: Describe the laboratory studies that show a combined role of learning and biology in the development of a fear reaction among Rhesus monkeys reared in a laboratory.

Answer: Monkeys raised in the lab show no fear of snakes. After watching adult monkeys exhibit fear reactions to snakes, the lab monkeys become fearful. However, the same process does not work when the lab monkeys watch other monkeys that appear to exhibit fear of rabbits. This suggests a selectivity factor, with the lab monkeys learning vicariously to fear only animals that they are "biologically wired" to fear (snakes, but not rabbits).

ES Moderate Page: 215 kind: c

6.122: Describe the hypothesized role of thought suppression in the etiology of obsessive-compulsive disorder.

Answer: Attempts to disregard or forget a troubling thought may actually make the thought more intrusive, as the troubling thought becomes associated with the other thoughts meant to replace it. The troubling thought also becomes associated with negative feelings, so that afterwards the negative feelings can trigger the unwanted thought, and the unwanted thought can trigger negative feelings.

ES Moderate Page: 219 kind: c

6.123: Describe Donald Klein's ideas on the hypothesized role of the suffocation response in the etiology of agoraphobia.

Answer: Agoraphobia may be triggered by a misfiring of cues alerting the body to increased levels of carbon dioxide or lactate. These cues lead to shortness of breath, and then to an alarm reaction as the body believes it is suffocating.

ES Moderate Page: 223 kind: c

Chapter 7
Maladaptive Responses to Stress

Multiple Choice Questions

7.1: Contemporary theories of the relation between
stress and illness hold that stress:

    a) is a factor in all physical illnesses, from the
       common cold to AIDS
    b) affects physical health but not psychological
       health
    c) affects psychological health but not physical
       health
    d) is influential in a limited number of diseases,
       such as ulcers

MC/Mod
Pg:236
kind:c
Ans:(a)

7.2: Current views of the etiology of physical illness:

    a) highlight the biological paradigm
    b) follow the biopsychosocial model
    c) incorporate humanistic concepts
    d) object to the diathesis-stress approach

MC/Mod
Pg:236
kind:c
Ans:(b)

7.3: Behavioral medicine is characterized by:

    a) the use of medication to control problem
       behaviors
    b) a focus on immunosuppression
    c) an emphasis on treating physical illness by
       changing behavior
    d) the use of behavior modification to treat
       psychological problems

MC/Mod
Pg:237
kind:c
Ans:(c)

7.4: Which of the following is an example of behavioral
medicine?

    a) lobotomy
    b) positive reinforcement for taking medications
    c) medications to control problem behaviors
    d) physical therapy to control pain

MC/Diff
Pg:237
kind:a
Ans:(b)

7.5: Which of the following problems is LEAST likely to be addressed in a behavioral medicine clinic?

a) a child refuses to wear orthopedic braces
b) a man with diabetes has a poor diet
c) a heart patient wants to stop smoking
d) an elderly woman mourns her husband

MC/Diff
Pg:237
kind:a
Ans:(d)

7.6: Health psychology is characterized by:

a) an emphasis on biological functioning rather than psychological functioning
b) a view of illness as an adaptive biological function
c) a concern with stress management, proper diet, and exercise
d) the study of the effects of stress on neurotransmitter production

MC/Easy
Pg:237
kind:c
Ans:(c)

7.7: Distress is defined as:

a) a unique cognitive appraisal of a stressor as stressful
b) the first step in coping with a stressor
c) a set of psychophysiological responses to stressors
d) the observable indicator of a stressor

MC/Mod
Pg:239
kind:f
Ans:(a)

7.8: A stressor is:

a) a negative emotional reaction
b) a trying event, irrespective of its effect on the individual
c) a psychophysiological reaction to an event
d) an individual's cognitive appraisal that something is trying

MC/Mod
Pg:239
kind:f
Ans:(b)

7.9: The most important criticism of the Social Readjustment Rating Scale is that it:

a) counts the number of stressors without taking into account how stressful each is
b) only looks at chronically stressful situations
c) applies mostly to college students
d) assumes that a given life event has the same consequences or meaning for all people

MC/Diff
Pg:240
kind:c
Ans:(d)

7.10: According to how the Social Readjustment Rating
Scale conceptualizes stress, an outstanding
personal achievement:

    a) can make up for stress in other areas
    b) is counted as stressful if it affects personal
       relationships
    c) is counted as stressful if it is unexpected,
       but not if expected
    d) is counted as stressful

7.11: Which of the following is an example of why some
researchers object to instruments like the Social
Readjustment Rating Scale?

    a) a stressor has a different meaning for
       different people
    b) a stressor doesn't necessarily affect social
       relationships
    c) a stressor can be a positive experience for
       some people
    d) a stressor doesn't necessarily cause immediate
       life changes

7.12: According to Richard Lazarus, what is the role of
cognition in stress?

    a) life events can be stressors even when not
       perceived as distressing
    b) life events are stressors only when perceived
       as distressing
    c) distress is an automatic cognitive reaction,
       independent of physiological reactions
    d) distress is an automatic physiological
       reaction, independent of cognitive reactions

7.13: Whose name is associated with the emergency
response?

    a) Lazarus   b) Seyle
    c) Cannon   d) Holmes

7.14: The emergency response as defined by Cannon is a:

    a) specific response depending on the stressor
    b) cognitive response or plan
    c) general arousal of the sympathetic nervous
       system
    d) tendency to flee from a strong stressor

MC/Mod
Pg:241
kind:c
Ans:(c)

7.15: Which of the following is typical of the emergency response?

    a) heart rate slows
    b) blood pressure drops
    c) blood sugar levels drop
    d) blood flows to muscles

MC/Easy
Pg:242
kind:f
Ans:(d)

7.16: According to Cannon, the purpose of the emergency response was to:

    a) slow the body down to avoid danger
    b) making thinking more clear in times of stress
    c) provide energy for sudden action
    d) scare predators or enemies

MC/Diff
Pg:242
kind:c
Ans:(c)

7.17: "Fight or flight" is associated with:

    a) the emergency response
    b) a cognitive appraisal of stress
    c) general adaptation syndrome
    d) arousal of the parasympathetic nervous system

MC/Mod
Pg:242
kind:c
Ans:(a)

7.18: Which of the following characterizes the "fight or flight" response?

    a) it is not evoked by psychological stressors
    b) it is most adaptive in the face of physically
       dangerous threats
    c) it is seen in other animals but not humans
    d) it is most adaptive in the face of
       psychological stressors

MC/Mod
Pg:242
kind:c
Ans:(b)

7.19: Which name is associated with the general adaptation syndrome?

    a) Cannon   b) Lazarus
    c) Seyle   d) Holmes

MC/Easy
Pg:242
kind:f
Ans:(c)

7.20: When an individual cannot respond to a threat with fight or flight or with other physical activity, which of the following occurs?

MC/Diff
Pg:242
kind:c
Ans:(d)

   a) the individual is prone to helplessness and depression
   b) the individual copes adaptively with more cognitive responses
   c) physiological reactions lessen and are replaced with psychological reactions
   d) physiological reactions are prolonged and maladaptive

7.21: According to Cannon, ongoing arousal of the sympathetic nervous system:

MC/Diff
Pg:242
kind:c
Ans:(c)

   a) maintains physical health
   b) regulates homeostasis
   c) is the link between stress and physical disorder
   d) is called the general adaptation syndrome

7.22: What are the stages of the general adaptation syndrome (GAS)?

MC/Mod
Pg:242
kind:c
Ans:(b)

   a) alertness, fight, flight
   b) alarm, resistance, exhaustion
   c) emergency response, general arousal, specific arousal
   d) general arousal, adaptation, homeostasis

7.23: In the general adaptation syndrome (GAS), the stage of resistance is:

MC/Mod
Pg:242
kind:c
Ans:(b)

   a) the "fight" aspect of fight or flight
   b) a period of physiological replenishment
   c) the individual's active decision to combat stress
   d) a period when the individual is least susceptible to stress

7.24: According to Seyle, the mechanism through which stress causes physical illness is:

MC/Diff
Pg:242
kind:c
Ans:(a)

   a) exhaustion
   b) the stage of alarm
   c) the stage of resistance
   d) the emergency response

7.25: The stress response is associated with lower levels of:

    a) adrenaline   b) epinephrine
    c) glucocorticoids   d) T-cells

MC/Mod
Pg:242
kind:c
Ans:(d)

7.26: Which of the following describes the process by which stress is thought to impair immune functioning?

    a) adrenal hormones inhibit T-cells
    b) adrenal hormones increase T-cells
    c) T-cells inhibit adrenal hormones
    d) T-cells increase adrenal hormones

MC/Mod
Pg:243
kind:f
Ans:(a)

7.27: Immunosuppression is characterized by decreased production of:

    a) mitogens   b) T-cells
    c) adrenal hormones d) red blood cells

MC/Mod
Pg:243
kind:c
Ans:(b)

7.28: Which is most important to the stress response?

    a) hippocampus
    b) parasympathetic nervous system
    c) adrenal gland
    d) lymphocytes

MC/Mod
Pg:243
kind:f
Ans:(c)

7.29: According to Dienstbier, a type of resilience called "physical toughness" can result from:

    a) intermittent mild or moderate stressors
    b) low or minimal stress
    c) frequent very challenging stressors
    d) use of the fight rather than the flight response

MC/Diff
Pg:243
kind:c
Ans:(a)

7.30: Recent researchers on stress differ from Seyle in that they have found:

a) different physiological responses to expected vs. unexpected stressors
b) different physiological responses to the fight vs. the flight response
c) a generalized response to stress, common to all stressors
d) lower, not higher glucocorticoids associated with stress

MC/Mod
Pg:244
kind:c
Ans:(a)

7.31: The most important distinction in types of coping that Lazarus and Folkman identified was:

a) nonspecific and specific
b) adaptive and maladaptive
c) emergency and resistance
d) problem-focused and emotion-focused

MC/Easy
Pg:244
kind:f
Ans:(d)

7.32: Earl works in an office where his office mate smokes. This irritates and frustrates Earl. Which of the following behaviors is an example of problem-focused coping?

a) using relaxation techniques to feel less frustrated
b) putting in a filter and opening a window
c) trying to see the office mate's point of view
d) thinking about the problem so much it interferes with work

MC/Mod
Pg:244
kind:a
Ans:(b)

7.33: Emotion-focused coping is:

a) an attempt to alter stress internally
b) an attempt to change a stressor
c) externally oriented
d) maladaptive

MC/Mod
Pg:244
kind:c
Ans:(a)

7.34: According to Folkman and Lazarus, when might emotion-focused coping be most effective?

a) when it is impossible to change the stressor
b) when the stressor is easily controlled
c) when problem-focused coping has already been effective
d) when the stressor is predictable

MC/Diff
Pg:244
kind:a
Ans:(a)

7.35: In an animal study of stress, a rat is given a   MC/Diff
       signal before being shocked. What is the effect of   Pg:245
       this signal?   kind:c
                                                             Ans:(c)

       a) the anticipation is more stressful than if
          there were no warning
       b) the anticipation leaves the rat in a
          chronically stressed state
       c) the anticipatory response is stressful, but
          weaker than if there were no warning
       d) the signal gives the rat a sense of a lack of
          control over the stressor

7.36: The 3 critical issues in cognitive responses to   MC/Diff
       stress are: Pg:245
                                                             kind:c
       a) alarm, resistance, exhaustion   Ans:(b)
       b) prediction, control, appraisal
       c) anticipation, repression, disclosure
       d) specificity, nonspecificity, problem-solving

7.37: Control can actually INCREASE stress when it is: MC/Diff
                                                             Pg:245
       a) perceived and can be exercised   kind:c
       b) illusory   Ans:(d)
       c) not predictable
       d) perceived but cannot be exercised

7.38: While walking through an abandoned area of town,   MC/Diff
       you hear a deafening alarm sounding from an empty   Pg:245
       warehouse. According to Folkman and Lazarus, under   kind:a
       which condition is this situation hypothesized to   Ans:(b)
       be most stressful?

       a) you know there is nothing you can do to stop
          the alarm
       b) you think you could stop the alarm if you could
          reach it, but you can't reach it
       c) you use emotion-focused coping before
          problem-focused coping
       d) you use problem-focused coping before
          emotion-focused coping

134

7.39: In a study of immunosuppression, students were assigned to 2 groups. One group wrote at length about a traumatic experience. The other group wrote at length about trivial experiences. Based on the results of this study, the researchers came to the general conclusion that talking about strong feelings:

MC/Diff
Pg:246
kind:c
Ans:(c)

    a) may change one's emotional state, but not one's physical state
    b) can increase immunosuppression
    c) may decrease stress-related illness
    d) may increase stress-related illness

7.40: The relationship between stress and physical illness is usually conceptualized as:

MC/Mod
Pg:247
kind:c
Ans:(c)

    a) unidirectional: stress worsens physical illness
    b) unidirectional: illness increases stress
    c) reciprocal: stress worsens illness and illness can be stressful
    d) unrelated except through immunosuppression

7.41: You are quite worried about final exams, concerned that you won't have enough credits. You find your stomach is upset and you have the dry heaves. This is an example of:

MC/Mod
Pg:248
kind:a
Ans:(d)

    a) a fictitious symptom
    b) a somatoform disorder
    c) immunosuppression
    d) a psychosomatic symptom

7.42: A psychosomatic illness is:

MC/Mod
Pg:248
kind:c
Ans:(b)

    a) an imaginary physical disorder
    b) a real physical disorder associated with psychological distress
    c) a fictitious psychological disorder
    d) a psychological, not physical illness

7.43: In the 1950s, psychoanalysts classified psychosomatic illnesses based on the specificity hypothesis. This held that:

    a) psychosomatic illness are caused by specific biological processes
    b) psychosomatic illnesses are caused by specific stressors
    c) only certain psychosomatic illnesses are pathological
    d) specific personality types cause specific psychosomatic disorders

MC/Diff
Pg:249
kind:c
Ans:(d)

7.44: In contrast to practitioners of psychosomatic medicine in the 1950s, contemporary researchers on psychosomatic illness:

    a) believe that all physical illnesses have psychological components
    b) believe that only certain physical illnesses have a psychological component
    c) believe in the specificity hypothesis
    d) call psychosomatic disorders "conversion disorders"

MC/Mod
Pg:249
kind:c
Ans:(a)

7.45: The essential integration of mind and body is highlighted in the DSM-IV by:

    a) a list of 10 "psychophysiological" disorders
    b) a separate diagnosis for medical conditions relevant to the treatment of emotional disorders
    c) a separate diagnosis for psychosomatic disorders
    d) introductory material noting that psychological experiences are critical in some physical illnesses

MC/Diff
Pg:249
kind:c
Ans:(b)

7.46: According to the threshold model of illness, "shell shock":

    a) only happens when there is brain damage from exploding artillery
    b) only happens to individuals with preexisting maladjustment
    c) can happen to anyone; everyone has a breaking point
    d) only happens when there is preexisting maladjustment and brain damage

MC/Mod
Pg:250
kind:c
Ans:(c)

136

7.47: In the DSM-IV, posttraumatic stress disorder (PTSD) is classified as:

a) an adjustment disorder
b) a psychosomatic illness
c) a psychosis
d) an anxiety disorder

MC/Mod
Pg:250
kind:f
Ans:(d)

7.48: An adjustment disorder is most likely to be associated with which of the following scenarios?

a) moving and getting a new job
b) a natural disaster
c) uncovering repressed memories of childhood trauma
d) ongoing anxiety after a car accident

MC/Diff
Pg:250
kind:a
Ans:(a)

7.49: Ratings of the severity of stressors in the DSM-III and DSM-III-R were abandoned in the DSM-IV because:

a) the list of possible stressors was too long
b) the guidelines for ratings were too detailed
c) the ratings showed low reliability
d) the number of stressors is more important than the severity

MC/Diff
Pg:251
kind:c
Ans:(c)

7.50: A major concern of behavioral medicine and health psychology is:

a) secondary hypertension
b) essential hypertension
c) diastolic hypertension
d) systolic hypertension

MC/Mod
Pg:252
kind:c
Ans:(b)

7.51: Which of the following exemplifies the relationship between stress and cardiovascular disease?

a) Type B personality is associated with higher blood pressure
b) stress is associated with poor health behaviors
c) stress is associated with thinned artery walls
d) stress causes people to focus on the warning signs of heart attack

MC/Diff
Pg:253
kind:c
Ans:(b)

137

7.52: The most stressful job situation is one which combines:

a) low decision control with low psychological demands
b) low decision control with high psychological demands
c) high decision control with low psychological demands
d) high decision control with high psychological demands

MC/Diff
Pg:254
kind:c
Ans:(b)

7.53: Social ecology refers to:

a) teaching people about pollution in the environment
b) the relationship between the individual and the social world
c) how human behaviors such as smoking contribute to pollution
d) maintaining a small group of close friends for social support

MC/Mod
Pg:256
kind:c
Ans:(b)

7.54: Which of the following characteristics of Type A behavior is most predictive of cardiovascular disease?

a) hostility
b) worrying
c) impatience
d) achievement orientation

MC/Mod
Pg:256
kind:c
Ans:(a)

7.55: A benefit of longitudinal research is that it:

a) is easier to conduct than cross sectional research
b) costs less than cross sectional research
c) allows one to rule out reverse causality
d) provides systematic control of stress

MC/Mod
Pg:257
kind:c
Ans:(c)

7.56: The retrospective method:

a) is a type of prospective design
b) may use public records to select subjects
c) is also known as a followup design
d) may ask subjects to recall past events

MC/Mod
Pg:257
kind:c
Ans:(d)

7.57: Which of the following characterizes the
      prospective research design?

      a) less subject to reporter bias than the
         retrospective design
      b) less effective than the retrospective design
      c) also known as the followback design
      d) also known as the cross-sectional design

MC/Mod
Pg:257
kind:c
Ans:(a)

7.58: An example of a primary prevention effort to reduce
      cardiovascular disease is:

      a) stress management for Type A behavior
      b) antismoking advertising for children
      c) biofeedback about blood pressure
      d) smoking cessation programs for cardiac patients

MC/Mod
Pg:258
kind:c
Ans:(b)

7.59: Biofeedback uses laboratory equipment to:

      a) provide relaxing stimuli to decrease blood
         pressure
      b) help the patient focus less on physiological
         processes
      c) lower blood pressure through relaxation
         training
      d) provide feedback about physical processes that
         are usually outside of awareness

MC/Mod
Pg:259
kind:c
Ans:(d)

7.60: As a treatment for hypertension, biofeedback:

      a) has found extensive research support
      b) has positive effects but only in the long term
      c) has not been supported by empirical evidence
      d) is only useful if medication is not being used

MC/Diff
Pg:259
kind:f
Ans:(c)

7.61: Relaxation training for patients with high blood
      pressure is an example of:

      a) primary prevention of coronary heart disease
      b) secondary prevention of coronary heart disease
      c) tertiary prevention of coronary heart disease
      d) treatment of coronary heart disease

MC/Mod
Pg:259
kind:c
Ans:(b)

7.62: Role playing can be effective in changing Type A behavior because:

a) patients get their frustrated feelings off their chest
b) patients understand what it feels like to be treated with hostility
c) the therapist models less hostile responses to frustration
d) participants confront each other about irrational thinking

MC/Mod
Pg:260
kind:c
Ans:(c)

7.63: Posttraumatic stress disorder (PTSD) is characterized by which of the following?

a) increased arousal of the sympathetic nervous system
b) re-experienced trauma and numbed emotional responses
c) decreases in arousal of the autonomic nervous system
d) development of alternate personalities

MC/Mod
Pg:260
kind:c
Ans:(b)

7.64: Posttraumatic stress disorder (PTSD) is classified as an anxiety disorder, but some psychologists believe it should be classified as:

a) an affective disorder
b) an adjustment disorder
c) a transient psychosis
d) a dissociative disorder

MC/Mod
Pg:261
kind:c
Ans:(d)

7.65: Most research on posttraumatic stress disorder (PTSD) has been on:

a) rape victims
b) victims of natural disaster
c) victims of sexual abuse
d) Vietnam war veterans

MC/Mod
Pg:261
kind:c
Ans:(d)

7.66: Adjustment disorders:

a) are not distressing
b) are caused by unusual stressors
c) are not considered to be mental disorders
d) are a form of posttraumatic stress disorder

MC/Mod
Pg:262
kind:c
Ans:(c)

7.67: Individuals with posttraumatic stress disorder (PTSD) also commonly meet the criteria for:

MC/Mod
Pg:263
kind:f
Ans:(b)

a) multiple personality disorder
b) depression and substance abuse
c) adjustment disorder with depressed mood
d) psychosis

7.68: Pre-existing psychological problems:

MC/Mod
Pg:263
kind:c
Ans:(a)

a) increase the risk for posttraumatic stress disorder
b) are unrelated to the risk for posttraumatic stress disorder
c) make it impossible to diagnose posttraumatic stress disorder
d) decrease the risk for posttraumatic stress disorder

7.69: Which of the following is true of posttraumatic stress disorder (PTSD)?

MC/Diff
Pg:265
kind:c
Ans:(c)

a) individuals with antisocial behavior are less likely to show PTSD
b) individuals with neurotic behaviors are less likely to show PTSD
c) family history of psychopathology is unrelated to PTSD in veterans exposed to high combat
d) family history of psychopathology is unrelated to PTSD in veterans exposed to low combat

7.70: An example of diathesis-stress in the development of posttraumatic stress disorder (PTSD) in war veterans is that veterans with premorbid adjustment problems:

MC/Mod
Pg:265
kind:c
Ans:(a)

a) are predisposed to PTSD even under low exposure to combat
b) only show PTSD if exposed to high levels of combat
c) tend to develop problems other than PTSD when exposed to combat
d) show the same rates of PTSD as veterans without premorbid adjustment problems

7.71: Some research links posttraumatic stress disorder   MC/Mod
with the combination of a poor premorbid   Pg:265
psychological adjustment and the experience of   kind:c
trauma. In this model: Ans:(d)

   a) premorbid personality and trauma are both
      diatheses
   b) premorbid personality and trauma are both
      stressors
   c) premorbid personality is a stressor, and trauma
      is a diathesis
   d) premorbid personality is a diathesis, and
      trauma is a stressor

7.72: Increased production of norepinephrine after trauma   MC/Diff
is associated with: Pg:265
                                                       kind:c
   a) more arousal, less aggression   Ans:(c)
   b) less arousal, more aggression
   c) more intense stress response
   d) less intense stress response

7.73: Trauma is hypothesized to affect which of the   MC/Mod
following?   Pg:265
                                                       kind:c
   a) decreases in norepinephrine   Ans:(c)
   b) destruction of new neural pathways
   c) increased endogenous opioids
   d) increased pain sensitivity

7.74: Psychoanalytic formulations of the symptoms of   MC/Diff
posttraumatic stress disorder (PTSD) focus on the   Pg:266
idea that: kind:c
                                                       Ans:(b)
   a) defense mechanisms exacerbate anxiety
   b) defense mechanisms lessen anxiety
   c) the specific defense mechanism used depends on
      the type of trauma experienced
   d) the content of flashbacks is interpretable

7.75: The two-factor theory explains the development of   MC/Mod
posttraumatic stress disorder (PTSD) following   Pg:266
trauma in terms of: kind:c
                                                       Ans:(d)
   a) reinforcement and punishment
   b) anxiety and phobias
   c) repression and withdrawal
   d) classical and operant conditioning

142

7.76: Learning theories of posttraumatic stress disorder (PTSD) hold that:

MC/Mod
Pg:266
kind:c
Ans:(d)

a) fear is paired with many other stimuli through operant conditioning
b) avoidance produces many fears through classical conditioning
c) only the unconditioned response is rational, not later conditioned responses
d) fear is maintained through avoidance

7.77: Evidence for the role of social support in the etiology of posttraumatic stress disorder (PTSD) is found in the example that Vietnam veterans:

MC/Mod
Pg:267
kind:c
Ans:(a)

a) did not receive social support on their return, and had high rates of PTSD
b) had high social support through the Veterans Administration, but still had high rates of PTSD
c) from closely knit units had lower rates of PTSD
d) from units that encouraged independence had lower rates of PTSD

7.78: Which of the following is thought to be important for emergency treatment after trauma?

MC/Diff
Pg:267
kind:c
Ans:(a)

a) the expectation that extreme distress is normal
b) getting the person away from the scene of the trauma
c) delaying treatment until the individual asks for help
d) expectation that the person probably won't have to re-experience the trauma

7.79: Which of the following is an important component of treating posttraumatic stress disorder (PTSD)?

MC/Mod
Pg:268
kind:c
Ans:(a)

a) re-experiencing the trauma in a controlled treatment setting
b) avoiding re-exposure to the trauma
c) emphasizing that the trauma is unrelated to other areas of life
d) reassurance that the trauma will not reoccur

7.80: In the treatment of posttraumatic stress disorder
(PTSD), desensitization is most helpful with
reducing:

    a) intrusive thoughts   b) avoidance
    c) nightmares   d) anger

MC/Mod
Pg:268
kind:c
Ans:(b)

True-False Questions

7.81: Psychological and emotional factors can affect
heart disease but not other diseases such as
diabetes.

TF/Easy
Pg:236
kind:f
Ans:False

7.82: Behavioral medicine relies on pharmaceutical
intervention to control problem behaviors.

TF/Mod
Pg:237
kind:f
Ans:False

7.83: Distress is the individual's physiological response
to a stressor.

TF/Easy
Pg:239
kind:c
Ans:False

7.84: Seyle was the first researcher who proposed the
idea that physical or psychological threats produce
general arousal of the sympathetic nervous system.

TF/Diff
Pg:241
kind:f
Ans:False

7.85: Seyle's idea of GAS refers to general arousal of
the sympathetic nervous system.

TF/Mod
Pg:242
kind:f
Ans:False

7.86: "Fight or flight" refers to the last stage of the
general adaptation syndrome.

TF/Mod
Pg:242
kind:c
Ans:False

7.87: Cannon proposed the idea that responses to stress
occur in 3 stages: alarm, resistance, and
exhaustion.

TF/Mod
Pg:242
kind:f
Ans:False

7.88: Trying to think differently about your mean boss is an example of emotion-focused coping.

TF/Mod
Pg:244
kind:c
Ans:True

7.89: Seyle's theory holds that the general adaptation syndrome (GAS) is activated in the same way by different stressors.

TF/Mod
Pg:244
kind:c
Ans:True

7.90: Cognitions can alter the stress response.

TF/Easy
Pg:245
kind:f
Ans:True

7.91: Psychosomatic illnesses are now known as somatoform illnesses.

TF/Mod
Pg:248
kind:f
Ans:False

7.92: A psychosomatic illness involves no real damage to the body.

TF/Mod
Pg:248
kind:f
Ans:False

7.93: Highest job strain is associated with high psychological demands and high decisional control.

TF/Diff
Pg:255
kind:c
Ans:False

7.94: Forms of emotional expression can contribute to the development of cardiovascular disease.

TF/Easy
Pg:256
kind:f
Ans:True

7.95: Type A personality is characterized by competitiveness and hostility.

TF/Mod
Pg:256
kind:c
Ans:True

7.96: The central Type A characteristic associated with cardiovascular disease is having high achievement goals.

TF/Mod
Pg:256
kind:f
Ans:False

7.97: Prospective longitudinal research is usually more expensive than retrospective longitudinal research.

TF/Mod
Pg:257
kind:f
Ans:True

7.98: Biofeedback and relaxation therapy are used to foster psychic numbing.

TF/Mod
Pg:259
kind:c
Ans:False

7.99: Posttraumatic stress disorder (PTSD) is classified as a dissociative disorder.

TF/Mod
Pg:261
kind:f
Ans:False

7.100: Adjustment disorder is used to diagnose an adverse reaction to an unusual event such as a natural disaster.

TF/Mod
Pg:262
kind:c
Ans:False

7.101: Trauma can affect biology by increasing the production of norepinephrine.

TF/Mod
Pg:265
kind:f
Ans:True

7.102: The 2-factor learning theory emphasizes the combination of a diathesis and a stressor.

TF/Mod
Pg:266
kind:c
Ans:False

Essay Questions

7.103: Describe the major benefit and the major drawback of defining stress in terms of stressors rather than in terms of subjective distress.

Answer: Benefit: can measure stress independent of its hypothesized effects.
Drawback: different people have different reactions to the same event.

ES Moderate Page: 239 kind: c

7.104: Explain the difference between Cannon's idea of the link between stress and physical disease and Seyle's idea of the link between stress and physical disease.

Answer: Seyle saw exhaustion as the link: after prolonged stress, the body can no longer respond appropriately and is subsequently damaged. Cannon saw chronic arousal as the link: experiencing "fight or flight" arousal, without being able to fight or flee, causes prolonged arousal of the sympathetic nervous system, which in turn causes physical damage to the body.

ES Moderate Page: 242 kind: c

7.105: Explain the difference between a psychosomatic disorder and a somatoform disorder.

Answer: A psychosomatic illness is a real physical illness with emotional or stress-related causes. A somatoform disorder has physical symptoms with no real physical damage, with purely psychological origins.

ES Moderate Page: 248 kind: c

7.106: Why are psychologists so interested in cardiovascular disease?

Answer: Psychologists can help change negative health behaviors such as smoking and low exercise. Also, personality styles and emotional expression affect CVD, which is a "lifestyle" disease.

ES Moderate Pages: 252-253 kind: c

7.107: Why do some researchers believe that posttraumatic stress disorder (PTSD) should be classified as a dissociative disorder rather than as an anxiety disorder?

Answer: PTSD often includes dissociative symptoms such as alterations in memory, alterations in consciousness, and reliving the trauma.

ES Moderate Page: 261 kind: c

Chapter 8
Dissociative and Somatoform Disorders

Multiple Choice Questions

8.1: The sudden onset of paralysis or blindness without
a clear biological cause is an example of:

    a) a dissociative disorder
    b) a somatoform disorder
    c) malingering
    d) depersonalization

MC/Easy
Pg:274
kind:f
Ans:(b)

8.2: What do dissociative and somatoform disorders have
in common?

    a) they have the same biological cause
    b) they both involve malingering
    c) they both involve unconscious processes
    d) people with these disorders also have
       personality disorders

MC/Mod
Pg:274
kind:c
Ans:(c)

8.3: Somatoform disorders are characterized by:

    a) no clear biological cause
    b) a known biological cause
    c) malingering
    d) purposeful presentation of impossible symptoms

MC/Easy
Pg:274
kind:f
Ans:(a)

8.4: Malingering means:

    a) unconscious dissociation of memory
    b) unintentional conversion of psychological
       symptoms
    c) loss of memory for one's identity
    d) pretending to have a problem or illness

MC/Easy
Pg:274
kind:f
Ans:(d)

8.5: Dissociative fugue shares some symptoms with other
dissociative disorders. However, the
DISTINGUISHING symptom of dissociative fugue is:

    a) inability to remember details of the past
    b) confusion about one's identity
    c) malingering
    d) purposeful, unplanned travel

MC/Mod
Pg:276
kind:f
Ans:(d)

8.6: The name "hysteria" is Greek for "wandering   MC/Mod
uterus." This name reflects the erroneous idea   Pg:277
that somatoform and dissociative disorders are   kind:c
caused by: Ans:(d)

a) gynecological dysfunction causing fevers
b) confused sexual identity
c) women misinterpreting mild symptoms as
catastrophic
d) women's frustrated desires to have children

8.7: Jean Charcot influenced the thinking of Freud as   MC/Mod
well as Freud's rival, Janet. Specifically, Freud   Pg:277
and Janet were influenced by Charcot's: kind:f
                                                        Ans:(d)
a) views on gynecology and psychopathology
b) integration of multiple personalities
c) discovery of biological causes of somatoform
disorders
d) use of hypnosis to treat and induce hysteria

8.8: Freud viewed dissociation as: MC/Mod
                                                        Pg:277
a) an abnormal process   kind:c
b) unlike repression   Ans:(c)
c) a routine expression of unconscious conflict
d) malingering

8.9: Janet viewed dissociation as: MC/Mod
                                                        Pg:277
a) a normal defense mechanism   kind:c
b) an abnormal process   Ans:(b)
c) malingering
d) similar to repression

8.10: As a result of Freudian influences, hysteria used MC/Mod
to be classified as a "neurosis," a category that   Pg:278
also included anxiety and depression. These were   kind:c
grouped together because: Ans:(d)

a) they are descriptively similar
b) they all involve memory impairment
c) they all involve identity disorder
d) unconscious conflict is seen as the common
cause

8.11: "Deja vu" experiences:

    a) are unrelated to dissociation
    b) are a sign of psychopathology
    c) can be eliminated with hypnosis
    d) are a normal form of dissociation

MC/Easy
Pg:278
kind:f
Ans:(d)

8.12: An anxious person at a crowded party suddenly feels as if he is a third person watching himself and the other people at the party. He is experiencing:

    a) deja vu   b) depersonalization
    c) identity disorder   d) fugue

MC/Mod
Pg:278
kind:a
Ans:(b)

8.13: Which of the following exemplifies the view of contemporary psychology regarding unconscious processes?

    a) they do not exist
    b) they are even more influential than Freud thought
    c) they are less influential than Freud thought
    d) they are only important in psychopathology

MC/Mod
Pg:278
kind:c
Ans:(c)

8.14: Psychogenic amnesia results from:

    a) emotional distress   b) brain injury
    c) brain disease   d) malingering

MC/Easy
Pg:279
kind:f
Ans:(a)

8.15: Which of the following typifies the course of recovery when amnesia or fugue follows a specific traumatic event?

    a) recovery is slow
    b) recovery is rapid
    c) recurrence is likely
    d) functioning rarely returns to normal

MC/Easy
Pg:279
kind:f
Ans:(b)

8.16: Lucinda witnesses a violent crime. Afterwards she cannot remember anything that happened before the trauma. This is called:

    a) posttraumatic amnesia
    b) anterograde amnesia
    c) retrograde amnesia
    d) selective amnesia

MC/Easy
Pg:279
kind:a
Ans:(c)

8.17: Rodney is involved in a near-death collision.   MC/Mod
Afterwards he cannot learn new information, such as   Pg:279
the name of his doctor in the hospital, what he   kind:a
ordered for lunch, and the time of his haircut   Ans:(d)
appointment. This is called:

a) retrograde amnesia
b) posttraumatic amnesia
c) selective amnesia
d) anterograde amnesia

8.18: The most common form of amnesia is: MC/Easy
                                                         Pg:279
a) retrograde amnesia   kind:f
b) posttraumatic amnesia   Ans:(c)
c) selective amnesia
d) anterograde amnesia

8.19: The association between trauma and a subsequent   MC/Mod
psychological disorder is clearest in the case of: Pg:279
                                                         kind:c
a) dissociative identity disorder   Ans:(b)
b) fugue
c) hysteria
d) somatoform disorder

8.20: A man is hypnotized to believe that his hand is   MC/Mod
numb. The hand is then placed in ice water, and   Pg:280
the man is able to leave his hand in the ice water   kind:c
for a long time, seemingly unaffected by pain.   Ans:(a)
However, when asked, the man can also describe the
pain that he does not appear to feel. This
phenomenon is known as:

a) hidden observer   b) psychogenic amnesia
c) suggestibility   d) somatoform disorder

8.21: Some psychologists do not see hypnosis as an   MC/Easy
altered state of consciousness. Rather, they see   Pg:280
being hypnotized as a: kind:c
                                                         Ans:(a)
a) response to suggestion and expectations
b) form of psychogenic amnesia
c) sign of predisposition to dissociation
d) form of depersonalization

8.22: Miller and Bowers (1986) conducted a study using subjects who had been classified as low or high in hypnotizability. Later, these subjects were either hypnotized or taught cognitive coping techniques to deal with pain. All subjects showed increased tolerance for pain, but there was also evidence that the effect was not just due to suggestion. Specifically, subjects in the "high hypnotizability" group showed the greater pain tolerance only when:

MC/Diff
Pg:280
kind:c
Ans:(a)

a) under hypnosis, not when in the cognitive coping group
b) in the cognitive coping group, not when under hypnosis
c) there was a hidden observer
d) there was no hidden observer

8.23: Depersonalization disorder is characterized by:

MC/Easy
Pg:281
kind:f
Ans:(a)

a) feeling as if you were in a dream or observing yourself
b) a rigid, delusional belief that you are not one person
c) a belief that you have multiple personalities
d) amnesia for your name and identity

8.24: Multiple personality disorder is also known as:

MC/Easy
Pg:281
kind:f
Ans:(c)

a) depersonalization
b) selective amnesia
c) dissociative identity disorder
d) dissociative fugue

8.25: The increase in diagnosis of multiple personality disorder in recent years has occurred in conjunction with:

MC/Mod
Pg:282
kind:f
Ans:(a)

a) recognition of the high prevalence of child sexual abuse
b) better assessment tools for diagnosis
c) increased use of hypnosis in therapy
d) more widespread drug use among teens

8.26: Some psychologists believe that the increase in the diagnosis of multiple personality disorder in recent years in the U.S. reflects a "fad." Support for this argument comes from evidence that:

MC/Mod
Pg:282
kind:f
Ans:(b)

a) there are more and more talk shows on this topic
b) the diagnosis is extremely rare in Japan and Europe
c) insurance companies will now cover treatment of multiple personality disorder
d) the diagnosis is made mostly by younger doctors

8.27: Not all psychologists agree that multiple personality disorder is a psychological disorder. The most commonly asserted alternative hypothesis used to explain behavior described as "multiple personality disorder" is that the patient:

MC/Mod
Pg:282
kind:c
Ans:(c)

a) has organic brain dysfunction
b) is under the influence of psychoactive drugs
c) responds to expectations by playing a role
d) has an affective disorder and mood swings

8.28: To test the role-playing hypothesis of multiple personality disorder, Spanos and colleagues have used what methodology?

MC/Mod
Pg:282
kind:c
Ans:(c)

a) induced hypnosis with patients
b) retrospective reports by therapists
c) analogue experiments in laboratories
d) diary studies with patients

8.29: To test the role-playing hypothesis of multiple personality disorder (MPD), Spanos and colleagues have conducted analogue experiments in which they asked college students to play the role of an accused murderer. The results of these studies showed that:

MC/Mod
Pg:283
kind:c
Ans:(c)

a) role playing causes multiple personality disorder
b) most subjects deny having a "hidden part", even under hypnosis
c) the symptoms of MPD can be induced through hypnosis
d) the ease of role-taking correlates with risk for MPD

8.30: Because of similar symptoms and etiology, some researchers have argued that dissociative disorders should be classified together with:

    a) posttraumatic stress disorder
    b) anxiety disorders
    c) affective disorders
    d) schizophrenia

MC/Diff
Pg:283
kind:c
Ans:(a)

8.31: Evidence that Kenneth Bianchi, the "Hillside Strangler," had multiple personality disorder was called into question because:

    a) the examiner asked leading questions
    b) Bianchi didn't know the names of the personalities
    c) Bianchi had low intelligence
    d) there was no known trauma in early life

MC/Mod
Pg:283
kind:c
Ans:(a)

8.32: Among the biological causes of dissociative STATES is:

    a) herpes   b) substance abuse
    c) pregnancy   d) Parkinson's disease

MC/Easy
Pg:284
kind:f
Ans:(b)

8.33: An individual with prosopagnosia:

    a) has multiple personalities
    b) cannot remember names
    c) has severe mood swings
    d) cannot recognize faces

MC/Easy
Pg:284
kind:f
Ans:(d)

8.34: Studies with patients with prosopagnosia show a dissociation between conscious and unconscious processes. Evidence for this phenomenon is that although patients claim not to be able to recognize faces:

    a) they prefer to look at pictures of strangers rather than familiar faces
    b) they prefer to look at pictures of familiar faces rather than strangers
    c) they can recognize voices
    d) they can recognize faces under hypnosis

MC/Mod
Pg:284
kind:c
Ans:(b)

8.35: Controversy about the role of trauma in the
etiology of multiple personality disorder is based
on:

a) case histories that show few cases associated
with trauma
b) poor reliability of the definition of trauma
c) concern about the validity of retrospective
reports
d) patients' hesitance to disclose trauma

MC/Mod
Pg:284
kind:c
Ans:(c)

8.36: Which of the following is an example of a
retrospective report?

a) a child describing what she expects high school
to be like
b) a teen describing how he likes high school
c) an adult describing what high school was like
d) evaluation of high school students' work by
several sources

MC/Easy
Pg:284
kind:f
Ans:(c)

8.37: Neisser and Harsch (1992) interviewed people about
how they learned about the explosion of the space
shuttle Challenger, and what they were doing at the
time. They interviewed people at the time of the
explosion, and then 3 years later. At the 3-year
followup:

a) nearly everyone showed accurate memories of
where they were
b) hardly anyone remembered what they were doing
c) leading questions led subjects to report false
memories
d) about 1/3 had vivid but inaccurate memories

MC/Mod
Pg:286
kind:f
Ans:(d)

8.38: An adequate test of the hypothesized relationship
between child abuse and dissociative disorder
requires:

a) retrospective analysis
b) intensive case studies of patients with
multiple personality disorder
c) accurate prevalence rates for child sexual
abuse
d) prospective research with objective measures

MC/Mod
Pg:286
kind:c
Ans:(d)

8.39: An example of state-dependent learning is that a   MC/Mod
person who learns something while she is happy: Pg:286
                                                           kind:a

a) will learn more quickly than if she is sad   Ans:(c)
b) will remember more than if she learned while
she was sad
c) will find it easier to remember what was
learned when she is happy again
d) will remember less than if she learned while
she was sad

8.40: Iatrogenesis refers to: MC/Mod
                                                          Pg:287

a) treatment causing, not curing, a disorder   kind:f
b) inability to recognize faces   Ans:(a)
c) emotional reliving of past experiences
d) state dependent learning

8.41: The emotional reliving of past traumatic   MC/Easy
experiences is called: Pg:287
                                                          kind:f

a) iatrogenesis   b) prosopagnosia   Ans:(d)
c) dissociation   d) abreaction

8.42: The main objective in treating multiple personality   MC/Easy
disorder is to: Pg:287
                                                          kind:c

a) induce amnesia for all but one personality   Ans:(b)
b) reintegrate the different personalities into a
whole
c) reduce depersonalization
d) stop abreaction

8.43: In contrast to psychosomatic disorder, the symptoms   MC/Easy
of somatoform disorder: Pg:288
                                                          kind:f

a) are due to an actual physical illness   Ans:(c)
b) make sense neurologically
c) cannot be explained by an underlying biological
problem
d) are unrelated to psychological factors

8.44: Theresa is unable to see, even though a physical examination shows no physical problems with her eyes or brain. She may be suffering from:

    a) psychosomatic disorder
    b) somatoform disorder
    c) dissociation
    d) fugue

MC/Mod
Pg:288
kind:a
Ans:(b)

8.45: A person with body dysmorphic disorder is likely to:

    a) have an imagined defect in his physical appearance
    b) have a strange body shape and associated low self-esteem
    c) show gastrointestinal problems when stressed
    d) show blindness or paralysis without physical cause

MC/Mod
Pg:288
kind:c
Ans:(a)

8.46: Unnecessary medical treatment is often associated with:

    a) psychosomatic illness
    b) somatoform disorder
    c) dissociative disorder
    d) amnesia

MC/Mod
Pg:288
kind:f
Ans:(b)

8.47: One problem associated with somatoform disorders is:

    a) organic brain dysfunction causing amnesia
    b) ulcers and stress-related illnesses
    c) legal difficulties due to having more than one personality
    d) high rates of unnecessary surgery

MC/Mod
Pg:289
kind:f
Ans:(d)

8.48: The preoccupation in body dysmorphic disorder usually focuses on:

    a) the nose and mouth   b) internal organs
    c) sense organs   d) the brain

MC/Easy
Pg:289
kind:f
Ans:(a)

8.49: The anxiety of hypochondriasis is:

    a) delusional in nature
    b) alleviated after a thorough physical examination
    c) not alleviated after a thorough physical evaluation
    d) associated with dissociation

MC/Mod
Pg:289
kind:c
Ans:(c)

8.50: A history of multiple somatic complaints in the absence of organic or biological problems is characteristic of:

    a) psychosomatic illness
    b) conversion disorder
    c) body dysmorphic disorder
    d) somatization

MC/Mod
Pg:290
kind:f
Ans:(d)

8.51: Patients with somatization disorder often present their symptoms in a histrionic manner. This means that they do so:

    a) in a vague but dramatic style
    b) with "la belle indifference"
    c) with gaps of memory
    d) in a way that makes no anatomical sense

MC/Mod
Pg:290
kind:f
Ans:(a)

8.52: A flippant lack of concern about symptoms, called "la belle indifference," is sometimes seen in patients with:

    a) pain disorder
    b) hypochondriasis
    c) somatization disorder
    d) psychosomatic illness

MC/Mod
Pg:290
kind:f
Ans:(c)

8.53: Some patients with somatization disorder show a flippant lack of concern about their physical symptoms. This is known as:

    a) histrionic style
    b) la belle indifference
    c) conversion
    d) dissociation

MC/Easy
Pg:290
kind:c
Ans:(b)

8.54: The symptoms of Briquet's syndrome are:

   a) hysterical blindness and paralysis
   b) multiple somatic complaints in the absence of organic problems
   c) imagined defects in bodily appearance
   d) dissociation and multiple personality

MC/Mod
Pg:290
kind:c
Ans:(b)

8.55: Briquet's syndrome is also known as:

   a) conversion disorder
   b) somatization disorder
   c) dissociative disorder
   d) body dysmorphic disorder

MC/Mod
Pg:290
kind:f
Ans:(b)

8.56: Pain disorder is a subtype of:

   a) dissociative disorder
   b) personality disorder
   c) psychosomatic disorder
   d) somatoform disorder

MC/Easy
Pg:290
kind:f
Ans:(d)

8.57: The symptoms of conversion disorder often resemble:

   a) gastrointestinal problems
   b) neurological impairments
   c) flu-like symptoms
   d) multiple personality disorder

MC/Easy
Pg:290
kind:f
Ans:(b)

8.58: Somatization disorder is much more common among:

   a) highly educated persons
   b) wealthy persons
   c) women
   d) men

MC/Mod
Pg:292
kind:f
Ans:(c)

8.59: Which of the following is equally common among women and men?

   a) somatization   b) conversion
   c) pain disorder   d) hypochondriasis

MC/Easy
Pg:292
kind:f
Ans:(d)

8.60: People who suffer from somatoform disorder also   MC/Mod
commonly suffer from: Pg:293
                                                             kind:c
a) dissociative disorder   Ans:(d)
b) schizophrenia
c) delusions
d) depression

8.61: Antisocial personality disorder is more common in   MC/Mod
men. A disorder that is thought to be related to   Pg:293
antisocial personality disorder but that is more   kind:f
common in women is: Ans:(d)

a) multiple personality disorder
b) eating disorders
c) sadistic personality disorder
d) somatization disorder

8.62: Often within one family, there will be one member   MC/Mod
with antisocial personality disorder and another   Pg:293
member with: kind:f
                                                            Ans:(a)
a) somatization disorder
b) pain disorder
c) conversion disorder
d) hypochondriasis

8.63: Antisocial personality disorder and somatization   MC/Diff
disorder are thought to be related in that they   Pg:293
both involve: kind:c
                                                            Ans:(a)
a) high negative emotion and the absence of
   inhibition
b) delusional thinking
c) dissociation
d) high demand for psychological treatment

8.64: A physical complaint is assumed to be part of a   MC/Easy
somatoform disorder when: Pg:293
                                                           kind:c
a) there is a history of other psychiatric   Ans:(d)
   problems
b) there are gaps in memory
c) the symptoms are gastrointestinal in nature
d) various known physical causes are ruled out

160

8.65: The diagnosis of somatoform disorder is sometimes mistakenly made in cases where there actually is an undetected physical illness. Typically, the eventual accurate diagnosis is a disorder such as:

MC/Mod
Pg:293
kind:f
Ans:(c)

a) ulcer or colitis
b) cardiovascular disease
c) epilepsy or multiple sclerosis
d) sensory deficits

8.66: In psychoanalytic theory, the symptoms of somatoform and dissociative disorders provide primary gain. This means that the symptoms:

MC/Mod
Pg:294
kind:c
Ans:(a)

a) protect the conscious mind from painful conflicts
b) allow benefits such as missing work
c) help the patient learn the sick role
d) are more easily treated than other problems

8.67: Marcy has a somatoform disorder. According to the cognitive behavioral perspective, her disorder is likely to be perpetuated by:

MC/Mod
Pg:294
kind:c
Ans:(a)

a) getting attention and getting to miss work
b) negative self-statements that reduce her self-esteem
c) complications from associated anxiety or depression
d) stigma from a society that labels her mentally ill

8.68: The cognitive behavioral idea that "learning the sick role" contributes to the etiology of somatoform disorders is LEAST instructive for:

MC/Mod
Pg:294
kind:c
Ans:(b)

a) pain disorder
b) conversion disorder
c) hypochondriasis
d) somatization disorder

8.69: Research on memory and retrospective reports shows that:

    a) depressed people erroneously recall more negative events
    b) anxiety is associated with long-term memory impairments
    c) specific memories are more reliable than global memories
    d) parents report more negative memories than children do

MC/Diff
Pg:295
kind:c
Ans:(c)

8.70: Many of Freud's patients who showed conversion disorder also described child sexual abuse. Although Freud later changed his mind, his EARLY conclusion was that:

    a) trauma causes conversion
    b) conversion precedes child abuse
    c) memories of sexual abuse are fantasies
    d) mental illness causes errors in memory

MC/Diff
Pg:296
kind:c
Ans:(a)

8.71: One theory about the lower prevalence of conversion disorders today as compared with 100 years ago is that today:

    a) there is less recreational cocaine use
    b) biological assessment is more accurate
    c) there is increased social acceptance of inner feelings
    d) psychoanalytic theory is less popular

MC/Mod
Pg:296
kind:c
Ans:(c)

8.72: The sociocultural view of the etiology of somatoform disorders suggests that these disorders are more common among nonindustrial societies and among the poorly educated in the U.S. because people in these communities:

    a) experience more pollution
    b) have less time to devote to introspection
    c) live in crowded conditions
    d) are suspicious of therapists

MC/Mod
Pg:296
kind:c
Ans:(b)

8.73: Operant behavioral approaches to treating chronic   MC/Mod
       pain are characterized by: Pg:296
                                                                 kind:f
       a) the use of pain as reinforcement   Ans:(c)
       b) the use of pain as punishment
       c) reduction in reinforcement for the sick role
       d) the use of biofeedback for relaxation

8.74: One reason for the limited research on the   MC/Easy
       psychological treatment of somatoform disorders is   Pg:296
       that most patients with somatoform disorders: kind:c
                                                                 Ans:(b)
       a) are of low intelligence
       b) see physicians, not psychologists
       c) improve without treatment
       d) dissociate too frequently to be assessed

8.75: The major recommendation for the medical management   MC/Mod
       of patients with somatoform disorder is: Pg:297
                                                                 kind:c
       a) medication to reduce anxiety   Ans:(b)
       b) a strong and consistent physician-patient
          relationship
       c) repeated medical procedures to reassure the
          patient
       d) confrontation of the patient's irrational
          thinking

True-False Questions

8.76: Dissociative disorders are characterized by   TF/Easy
       disruptions in the integration of memory,   Pg:274
       consciousness, or identity.   kind:f
                                                                 Ans:True

8.77: Dissociative fugue is usually not associated with   TF/Easy
       any specific event or trauma.   Pg:276
                                                                 kind:f
                                                                 Ans:False

8.78: An early diagnostic category that is no longer used   TF/Easy
       was "hysteria." This category included somatoform   Pg:277
       and dissociative disorders.   kind:f
                                                                 Ans:True

163

8.79: Jean Charcot influenced the thinking of Freud as well as Freud's rival Janet.

TF/Easy
Pg:277
kind:f
Ans:True

8.80: In contrast to Freud, contemporary scientists view unconscious events as much less influential in shaping behavior.

TF/Easy
Pg:278
kind:f
Ans:True

8.81: Psychogenic amnesia results from brain injury.

TF/Easy
Pg:279
kind:f
Ans:False

8.82: Depersonalization involves a rigid, delusional belief that one is living in a dream or floating outside of one's body.

TF/Easy
Pg:281
kind:f
Ans:False

8.83: The onset of depersonalization disorder often follows a new or disturbing event such as drug use.

TF/Easy
Pg:281
kind:f
Ans:True

8.84: The prevalence of dissociative disorders is difficult to establish, but the conditions generally have been considered to be extremely rare.

TF/Easy
Pg:282
kind:f
Ans:True

8.85: Dissociative disorders are often precipitated by trauma.

TF/Easy
Pg:283
kind:f
Ans:True

8.86: If the cause of a dissociative state is substance abuse, the diagnosis of dissociative disorder is not made, according to DSM-IV criteria.

TF/Mod
Pg:284
kind:f
Ans:True

8.87: Few people can report accurate memories from before age 3 or 4.

TF/Easy
Pg:285
kind:f
Ans:True

8.88: The central aspect of treating dissociative disorders is helping the patient to forget past traumatic events.

TF/Mod
Pg:287
kind:c
Ans:False

8.89: There has been little systematic research on the effectiveness of treatments for dissociative disorders.

TF/Easy
Pg:287
kind:f
Ans:True

8.90: The symptoms of somatoform disorders are due to actual physical illnesses associated with stress.

TF/Mod
Pg:288
kind:f
Ans:False

8.91: Somatization disorder usually begins in middle age.

TF/Mod
Pg:290
kind:f
Ans:False

8.92: The central assumption of conversion disorder is that physical illnesses cause psychological conflicts.

TF/Mod
Pg:291
kind:c
Ans:False

8.93: According to psychoanalytic theory, the symptoms of somatoform and dissociative disorders provide secondary gain. A cognitive behavioral term for this is reinforcement.

TF/Easy
Pg:294
kind:f
Ans:True

8.94: Conversion disorders are much more rare today than they were in Freud's time.

TF/Easy
Pg:296
kind:f
Ans:True

8.95: Somatoform disorders are more common in industrialized societies.

TF/Easy
Pg:296
kind:f
Ans:False

Essay Questions

8.96: Describe the characteristics of dissociative fugue, which provide evidence that the mind possesses different levels of consciousness.

Answer: An individual in a fugue state is aware of the present, has a purpose in going somewhere, and yet is unaware of the past. The individual loses only parts of awareness.

ES   Moderate   Page: 276   kind: c

8.97: Recovered memories from early childhood have become an important and controversial issue. Discuss the reasons for this controversy and the research evidence that casts doubt on some reports of "recovered memories."

Answer: (1) Memory research indicates that most memories from preschool are forgotten. (2) Therapists rarely doubt their patients' memories and may ask leading questions or set up expectations that induce false memories. (3) Research indicates high rates of erroneous memories for important events, such as where people were on the day the space shuttle Challenger blew up.

ES   Difficult   Pages: 285-286   kind: c

8.98: Explain how the phenomenon of state dependent learning has been used to explain multiple personality disorder.

Answer: (1) Experiences in a dissociated state are most easily recalled when dissociating. (2) Repeated trauma, dissociation, and state dependent learning lead to more complete and autonomous memories. (3) Independent personalities develop that dominate during different states of consciousness.

ES   Moderate   Page: 286   kind: c

8.99: Describe the association between antisocial personality disorder and somatization disorder.

Answer: (1) Often co-occur in the same family, but not the same individual. (2) Similar course: early onset, chronic, low SES groups. (3) Similar associated problems: substance abuse, marital problems, suicidality. (4) High negative emotion, low inhibition.

ES   Difficult   Page: 293   kind: c

166

8.100: Explain the cognitive behavioral perspective on the role of learning in the etiology of somatoform disorders.

Answer: (1) Caused by learning the sick role. (2) Secondary gain through reinforcement for sick behaviors. (3) Positive reinforcement through attention; negative reinforcement through avoiding work; modeling.

ES Moderate Page: 294 kind: c

Chapter 9
Personality Disorders

Multiple Choice Questions

9.1: Someone with a personality disorder shows behavior that is:

    a) more impaired than that associated with most other mental disorders
    b) rigid and inflexible
    c) problematic off and on, not chronically
    d) clustered

MC/Easy
Pg:302
kind:c
Ans:(b)

9.2: There is disagreement about what behaviors constitute a personality disorder. For example, 2 types of personality disorder in the U.S. system (DSM-IV) are not included in the European system (ICD-10). These 2 personality disorders are:

    a) avoidant and antisocial
    b) histrionic and dependent
    c) borderline and schizotypal
    d) paranoid and schizoid

MC/Mod
Pg:302
kind:f
Ans:(c)

9.3: One reason that personality disorders are controversial is that they:

    a) are difficult to diagnose reliably
    b) were conceptualized for insurance purposes
    c) are not associated with social or occupational problems
    d) are easily learned and unlearned, and so don't require therapy

MC/Mod
Pg:302
kind:c
Ans:(a)

9.4: In the DSM-IV system of diagnosis, personality disorders are listed on Axis:

    a) I   b) II
    c) III   d) IV

MC/Easy
Pg:302
kind:f
Ans:(b)

9.5: Most forms of mental disorder are "ego dystonic."
This means that people with these disorders:

a) have underdeveloped ego functions
b) lack a clear sense of identity
c) do not see themselves as having a problem
d) are distressed by their symptoms

MC/Mod
Pg:305
kind:c
Ans:(d)

9.6: Temperament refers to:

a) remorse over doing something wrong
b) insight into one's problems
c) anger over abandonment or loss
d) a behavioral style evident early in life

MC/Mod
Pg:306
kind:c
Ans:(d)

9.7: Which of the following is thought to contribute to
a person's temperament?

a) feelings of guilt
b) activity level and irritability
c) ego development
d) personality development

MC/Easy
Pg:306
kind:c
Ans:(b)

9.8: Unlike temperament, the concept of personality
includes a consideration of:

a) genetics
b) intelligence
c) others' reactions
d) coping and motivational factors

MC/Mod
Pg:306
kind:c
Ans:(d)

9.9: The long-term impact of a child's temperament
depends on:

a) how easy-going the child is
b) how intelligent the child is
c) how unusual it is
d) how it fits with the environment and is
   interpreted

MC/Mod
Pg:307
kind:c
Ans:(d)

9.10: One fundamental assumption of most personality theories is the notion that a person's behavior is:

    a) determined by genetics
    b) entirely learned
    c) understood best by the individual, not an observer
    d) stable across time and across situations

MC/Mod
Pg:307
kind:c
Ans:(d)

9.11: The social learning position on the person-situation debate is that behavior is determined by:

    a) internal personality traits
    b) the context in which it occurs
    c) genetics
    d) free will

MC/Mod
Pg:307
kind:c
Ans:(b)

9.12: One method employed to improve the procedures used to identify stable personality traits has been:

    a) counting the frequency of specific behaviors
    b) rating general response styles
    c) observing behavior at 1 or 2 isolated moments
    d) asking people about their own personality

MC/Mod
Pg:308
kind:c
Ans:(b)

9.13: Descriptions of personality traits show the highest reliability when behavior is observed:

    a) on repeated occasions
    b) on one occasion
    c) in a laboratory setting
    d) at an early age

MC/Easy
Pg:308
kind:f
Ans:(a)

9.14: In personality theory, neuroticism refers to:

    a) bizarre and unusual thinking
    b) expression of anxiety and depression
    c) low interest in interacting with other people
    d) conscientiousness

MC/Easy
Pg:309
kind:f
Ans:(b)

9.15: The 3 "clusters" of personality disorder in the DSM-IV were derived on the basis of:

a) empirical evidence of co-morbidity
b) empirical evidence of genetic relatedness
c) the various disorders' prevalence
d) intuition about their similarity

MC/Mod
Pg:310
kind:f
Ans:(d)

9.16: The paranoid, schizoid, and schizotypal personality disorders are all thought to be behavioral traits or interpersonal styles that:

a) follow a schizophrenic episode
b) are commonly mistaken for schizophrenia
c) sometimes precede onset of a full-blown psychosis
d) are unrelated to schizophrenia

MC/Easy
Pg:310
kind:c
Ans:(c)

9.17: Schizoid personality disorder is often characterized by:

a) unusual perceptual experiences
b) inappropriate suspiciousness
c) psychosis
d) indifference to other people

MC/Mod
Pg:310
kind:c
Ans:(d)

9.18: Schizotypal personality disorder is characterized by:

a) unusual perceptual experiences
b) indifference to other people
c) inappropriate suspiciousness
d) psychosis

MC/Mod
Pg:310
kind:c
Ans:(a)

9.19: Antisocial personality disorder is characterized by:

a) irresponsible behavior and lack of guilt
b) disinterest in human relationships
c) peculiar thinking
d) psychosis

MC/Easy
Pg:311
kind:f
Ans:(a)

171

9.20: The antisocial behavior associated with antisocial
      personality disorder:

      a) is by definition criminal in nature
      b) begins in childhood or adolescence
      c) goes away in adulthood
      d) begins in adulthood

MC/Easy
Pg:311
kind:c
Ans:(b)

9.21: Instability of mood, intense and unstable
      relationships, and difficulty being alone are all
      characteristic of:

      a) borderline personality disorder
      b) schizoid personality disorder
      c) antisocial personality disorder
      d) avoidant personality disorder

MC/Easy
Pg:312
kind:c
Ans:(a)

9.22: Exaggerated emotionality and attention-seeking are
      core characteristics of:

      a) histrionic personality disorder
      b) obsessive-compulsive personality disorder
      c) schizotypal personality disorder
      d) antisocial personality disorder

MC/Easy
Pg:313
kind:c
Ans:(a)

9.23: Narcissistic personality disorder is characterized
      by an exaggerated:

      a) sense of self-importance
      b) intensity in close relationships
      c) emotionality
      d) feeling of social anxiety

MC/Mod
Pg:313
kind:c
Ans:(a)

9.24: Kelly has been diagnosed as having avoidant
      personality disorder. She dislikes going to
      parties and is very anxious when unsure of what
      will happen in social situations. This is likely
      to be because Kelly:

      a) is disinterested in other people
      b) is preoccupied with rules
      c) wants to be the center of attention
      d) wants to be liked but is afraid of criticism

MC/Mod
Pg:313
kind:a
Ans:(d)

9.25: A person with dependent personality disorder and a
      person with avoidant personality disorder are both
      likely to:

      a) seek advice and reassurance
      b) avoid closeness
      c) be sensitive and easily hurt by criticism
      d) be preoccupied with rules

MC/Diff
Pg:313
kind:c
Ans:(c)

9.26: Perfectionism is a core trait of:

      a) obsessive-compulsive personality disorder
      b) histrionic personality disorder
      c) antisocial personality disorder
      d) avoidant personality disorder

MC/Mod
Pg:314
kind:c
Ans:(a)

9.27: Unlike obsessive-compulsive personality disorder,
      obsessive-compulsive disorder involves:

      a) dependency and advice-seeking
      b) excessive emotionality
      c) intrusive thoughts and ritualistic behavior
      d) lack of guilt

MC/Mod
Pg:314
kind:c
Ans:(c)

9.28: In the 5-factor model of personality, the dimension
      of conscientiousness is most related to the
      category that DSM-IV calls:

      a) histrionic personality disorder
      b) borderline personality disorder
      c) obsessive-compulsive personality disorder
      d) schizoid personality disorder

MC/Mod
Pg:315
kind:f
Ans:(c)

9.29: The DSM-IV method, which classifies personality
      disorders as discrete categories rather than
      dimensional, traits has been criticized because:

      a) labels created more problems than they solve
      b) a categorical approach does not explain
         etiology
      c) one category usually does not adequately
         describe a person
      d) the category names are arbitrary

MC/Mod
Pg:315
kind:c
Ans:(c)

9.30: Borderline, narcissistic, and histrionic personality disorder are all characterized by high levels of which trait?

   a) extraversion   b) agreeableness
   c) conscientiousness d) openness

MC/Mod
Pg:315
kind:c
Ans:(a)

9.31: Which of the following personality disorders is associated with high levels of the trait of "agreeableness"?

   a) paranoid   b) borderline
   c) narcissistic   d) dependent

MC/Mod
Pg:315
kind:c
Ans:(d)

9.32: In terms of trait descriptions, obsessive-compulsive personality disorder is defined in terms of high:

   a) conscientiousness b) openness
   c) agreeableness   d) extraversion

MC/Mod
Pg:315
kind:c
Ans:(a)

9.33: The Schedule for Nonadaptive and Adaptive Personality (SNAP) is a personality inventory that is characterized by:

   a) categorical descriptions similar to the DSM-IV
   b) a semi-structured interview format
   c) descriptions of 3 clusters of personality disorder
   d) descriptions of traits on 12 dimensions

MC/Mod
Pg:316
kind:c
Ans:(d)

9.34: A researcher is studying antisocial personality disorder and decides to use a paper and pencil self-report inventory asking about behaviors associated with this diagnosis. The researcher's estimate of the rate of antisocial personality disorder in the sample is likely to be:

   a) an overestimate
   b) accurate
   c) an underestimate
   d) the same as if interviews were conducted

MC/Mod
Pg:316
kind:a
Ans:(c)

9.35: The lifetime prevalence of personality disorders in
the U.S. is about:

    a) 3%   b) 12%
    c) 34%   d) 52%

MC/Mod
Pg:316
kind:f
Ans:(b)

9.36: The rarest personality disorders in the U.S. are
thought to be:

    a) borderline and obsessive-compulsive
    b) histrionic and schizotypal
    c) avoidant and dependent
    d) schizoid and narcissistic

MC/Diff
Pg:316
kind:f
Ans:(d)

9.37: The prevalence of antisocial personality disorder
is likely to be highest in a population of:

    a) hospitalized psychiatric patients
    b) outpatient therapy clients
    c) prison inmates
    d) children

MC/Easy
Pg:317
kind:f
Ans:(c)

9.38: A personality disorder that has little overlap with
others is:

    a) histrionic
    b) obsessive-compulsive
    c) borderline
    d) schizotypal

MC/Mod
Pg:317
kind:c
Ans:(b)

9.39: Conduct disorder in children (especially males) is
a predictor of what disorder in adulthood?

    a) antisocial personality disorder
    b) avoidant personality disorder
    c) schizotypal personality disorder
    d) narcissistic personality disorder

MC/Easy
Pg:317
kind:f
Ans:(a)

9.40: The most common personality disorder found among
persons in inpatient and outpatient treatment
settings is:

    a) antisocial personality disorder
    b) borderline personality disorder
    c) dependent personality disorder
    d) schizotypal personality disorder

MC/Mod
Pg:317
kind:f
Ans:(b)

9.41: In adolescents, personality disorders are:

    a) rare and unstable
    b) prevalent and unstable
    c) rare and stable
    d) prevalent and stable

MC/Mod
Pg:318
kind:c
Ans:(b)

9.42: Among patients who have received professional treatment for their problems, the long-term prognosis is especially poor among persons with:

    a) borderline personality disorder
    b) avoidant personality disorder
    c) obsessive-compulsive personality disorder
    d) schizoid personality disorder

MC/Mod
Pg:318
kind:c
Ans:(d)

9.43: Some critics contend that certain personality disorder diagnoses are sexist labels. In these cases, these critics believe that behavior called "pathological" in women is actually:

    a) a manifestation of gynecological problems
    b) a way of coping with oppressive circumstances
    c) a representation of different value systems
    d) feminine behavior that is threatening to male clinicians

MC/Mod
Pg:318
kind:c
Ans:(b)

9.44: Many men with histrionic personality disorder also have:

    a) identity disorder
    b) substance abuse disorder
    c) sexual problems
    d) adjustment disorder

MC/Easy
Pg:319
kind:f
Ans:(b)

9.45: A disorder that is 6 times more common in men than in women is:

    a) avoidant personality disorder
    b) narcissistic personality disorder
    c) antisocial personality disorder
    d) schizotypal personality disorder

MC/Easy
Pg:320
kind:f
Ans:(c)

9.46: A diagnostic category that is heavily influenced by psychodynamic theories about the origins of personality traits is:

MC/Mod
Pg:320
kind:c
Ans:(b)

    a) obsessive-compulsive personality disorder
    b) borderline personality disorder
    c) schizotypal personality disorder
    d) antisocial personality disorder

9.47: "Simple schizophrenia" was a term used in the 1960s to describe what DSM-IV now calls:

MC/Mod
Pg:320
kind:c
Ans:(a)

    a) schizoid personality traits
    b) a first episode of schizophrenia
    c) hallucinations without delusions
    d) delusions without hallucinations

9.48: In 1980, DSM-III put avoidant personality disorder in a separate category from schizotypal, schizoid, and paranoid personality disorders based on the idea that avoidant personality disorder involves more:

MC/Mod
Pg:321
kind:c
Ans:(c)

    a) social isolation
    b) indifference to other people
    c) expressed anxiety
    d) flamboyance

9.49: Family studies have demonstrated that the first-degree relatives of schizophrenic patients:

MC/Mod
Pg:321
kind:f
Ans:(c)

    a) rarely show schizotypal personality disorder
    b) almost always show schizotypal personality disorder
    c) show higher than average rates of schizotypal personality disorder
    d) show lower than average rates of schizotypal personality disorder

9.50: Children of parents with schizophrenia often show schizotypal personality disorder. This is also frequently true of children whose parents have:

MC/Mod
Pg:321
kind:f
Ans:(b)

    a) substance abuse disorder
    b) mood disorder
    c) antisocial personality disorder
    d) histrionic personality disorder

9.51: Many schizophrenic patients and their first degree   MC/Mod
relatives show impairment in: Pg:322
                                                              kind:c
a) hearing and auditory discrimination   Ans:(c)
b) tactile accuracy
c) smooth pursuit eye movements
d) motor coordination

9.52: Generally, personality disorders are ego syntonic   MC/Mod
in nature. This means that the patient: Pg:323
                                                              kind:c
a) is distressed by and perhaps ashamed of the   Ans:(d)
   problem
b) often suffers other disorders as well
c) has very high insight into the problem
d) does not see the disorder as a problem

9.53: One problem in treating personality disorder   MC/Easy
patients is: Pg:323
                                                              kind:c
a) high drop out rate   Ans:(a)
b) high distress about problems
c) low intelligence
d) related physical problems

9.54: According to Kernberg, the common characteristic of   MC/Easy
people with borderline personality disorder is: Pg:323
                                                              kind:c
a) impaired smooth pursuit eye movements   Ans:(c)
b) lack of guilt
c) faulty development of ego structure
d) preoccupation with rules

9.55: Psychodynamic theorists have argued that borderline   MC/Mod
personality disorder is related to underdeveloped: Pg:323
                                                              kind:c
a) ego structure   Ans:(a)
b) id
c) superego
d) primary process thinking

178

9.56: According to Kernberg, people with borderline   MC/Mod
       personality disorder often engage in primary   Pg:324
       process thinking. This means: kind:c
                                                            Ans:(a)
       a) imagining that what one wants is actually true
       b) seeing people as all good or all bad
       c) being ruled by one's emotions
       d) manipulating others' words to avoid feeling
          guilty

9.57: "Splitting" by a borderline personality disorder   MC/Mod
       patient refers to: Pg:324
                                                            kind:c
       a) lack of impulse control   Ans:(b)
       b) seeing people as all good or all bad
       c) imagining that what one wants is actually true
       d) brain dysfunction causing attention deficit

9.58: A borderline personality disorder patient sees his   MC/Mod
       girlfriend as "the most perfect person in the   Pg:324
       world" when she brings him a present, but is   kind:a
       enraged and sees her as "an evil jerk" when she has Ans:(a)
       to leave his birthday party early. This behavior
       is characteristic of borderline personality
       disorder and is known as:

       a) splitting
       b) primary process thinking
       c) poor impulse control
       d) ego dystonia

9.59: Akiskal contends that the category of borderline   MC/Mod
       personality disorder is not a valid or meaningful   Pg:324
       diagnostic concept because the symptoms are: kind:c
                                                            Ans:(a)
       a) heterogeneous and associated with many other
          disorders
       b) too mild to be classified as pathological
       c) easily learned and unlearned
       d) too transient to be classified as pathological

9.60: A disorder that commonly co-occurs with borderline   MC/Easy
       personality disorder is: Pg:324
                                                            kind:f
       a) depression   Ans:(a)
       b) generalized anxiety disorder
       c) phobia
       d) schizophrenia

179

9.61: Early loss or unavailability of a parent figure is thought to contribute to the etiology of:

MC/Mod
Pg:325
kind:c
Ans:(c)

    a) schizophrenia
    b) phobias
    c) borderline personality disorder
    d) obsessive-compulsive personality disorder

9.62: Borderline personality disorder is especially difficult to treat with psychotherapy because patients with this disorder:

MC/Mod
Pg:326
kind:c
Ans:(d)

    a) are generally of very low intelligence
    b) are indifferent to others
    c) are psychotic and need medication
    d) have trouble forming a close relationship with the therapist

9.63: Dialectical behavior therapy with borderline personality disorder patients combines behavior therapy techniques with:

MC/Mod
Pg:327
kind:c
Ans:(a)

    a) supportive and accepting psychotherapy
    b) psychotropic medication
    c) electroconvulsive therapy
    d) education for family members

9.64: The personality disorder that has been studied the most thoroughly and for the longest period of time is:

MC/Mod
Pg:327
kind:c
Ans:(d)

    a) schizotypal personality disorder
    b) histrionic personality disorder
    c) borderline personality disorder
    d) antisocial personality disorder

9.65: "Moral insanity" and "psychopathic insanity" are both terms used in the 19th century to describe what is today called:

MC/Easy
Pg:327
kind:f
Ans:(b)

    a) borderline personality disorder
    b) antisocial personality disorder
    c) schizoid personality disorder
    d) obsessive-compulsive personality disorder

9.66: Which of the following characterizes psychopathy as described by Cleckley (1941)?

    a) psychotic, delusional, schizoid
    b) has mood swings, dependent, anxious
    c) impulsive, self-centered, lacks guilt
    d) confused sexual identity, guilt-ridden, impotent

MC/Mod
Pg:327
kind:c
Ans:(c)

9.67: In the DSM-III, the description of antisocial personality disorder (ASP) was made more reliable by focusing on tangible consequences of antisocial personality traits, such as failure to conform to social norms with respect to lawful behavior. This approach was modified in DSM-IV because the critics thought that DSM-III's description of ASP:

    a) focused too much on the lack of remorse
    b) blurred the distinction between criminality and ASP
    c) did not take into account substance abuse
    d) relied too much on the presence of childhood conduct disorder

MC/Mod
Pg:328
kind:c
Ans:(b)

9.68: A common co-occurring problem in persons with antisocial personality disorder is:

    a) psychosis
    b) substance abuse
    c) anxiety disorder
    d) obsessive-compulsive personality disorder

MC/Easy
Pg:328
kind:f
Ans:(b)

9.69: Long-term studies of antisocial behavior in psychopaths suggest that these behaviors:

    a) increase over time throughout adulthood
    b) remain constant throughout adulthood
    c) eventually decrease in middle age
    d) rarely begin in childhood

MC/Mod
Pg:328
kind:c
Ans:(c)

9.70: Studies of antisocial personality disorder in biological and adoptive families have focused mostly on:

    a) arrest records and criminal behavior
    b) lack of remorse or guilt
    c) thrill-seeking behavior
    d) impulse control

MC/Mod
Pg:330
kind:c
Ans:(a)

9.71: Studies of antisocial personality disorder in
      biological and adoptive families have found that
      the highest rates of criminality are found in
      children:

      a) whose biological parent is a criminal
      b) whose adoptive parent is a criminal
      c) whose biological and adoptive parents both show
         criminality
      d) who undergo multiple adoptions

MC/Easy
Pg:330
kind:f
Ans:(c)

9.72: Seeking high levels of stimulation is a trait
      characteristic of:

      a) schizotypal personality disorder
      b) avoidant personality disorder
      c) antisocial personality disorder
      d) obsessive-compulsive personality disorder

MC/Mod
Pg:330
kind:f
Ans:(c)

9.73: In laboratory studies, subjects are asked to learn
      a sequence of responses in order to receive a
      reward or punishment. When psychopaths are
      compared to nonpsychopaths, it is found that
      psychopaths:

      a) have a much more difficult time learning
      b) show high aversion to anticipated punishment
      c) show high intelligence and better performance
      d) do not seem to experience anticipated
         punishment as aversive

MC/Mod
Pg:331
kind:c
Ans:(d)

9.74: Most antisocial behavior seen during adolescence:

      a) is a sign of antisocial personality disorder
      b) disappears in adulthood
      c) is a continuation of behavior problems seen in
         childhood
      d) predicts later criminality

MC/Mod
Pg:332
kind:c
Ans:(b)

9.75: Moffitt classifies antisocial behavior as "lifecourse-persistent" and "adolescence-limited." Which of the following typifies the lifecourse-persistent category?

    a) equal numbers of women and men
    b) much more common than adolescence-limited antisocial behavior
    c) expressed through different problem behaviors at different ages
    d) rarely associated with antisocial personality disorder

MC/Mod
Pg:332
kind:f
Ans:(c)

9.76: Studies have found that children and adolescents who engage in persistently antisocial behavior often show subtle deficits on neuropsychological tests in the area of "executive functions." Executive functions are related to:

    a) intelligence
    b) reading and verbal reasoning
    c) job skills
    d) impulse control

MC/Mod
Pg:332
kind:c
Ans:(d)

9.77: According to Moffitt, the subtle neurological problems in children who show antisocial behavior are presumably expressed in the form of:

    a) mental retardation
    b) neuroticism
    c) difficult temperament
    d) sensory impairments

MC/Mod
Pg:332
kind:f
Ans:(c)

9.78: The success of psychological treatment for antisocial personality disorder is generally:

    a) very high
    b) very limited
    c) lower when there is also depression
    d) higher when family members are involved

MC/Mod
Pg:333
kind:c
Ans:(b)

True-False Questions

9.79: Most people with personality disorders seek professional help.

TF/Easy
Pg:302
kind:f
Ans:False

9.80: The personality disorders are conceptualized in DSM-IV as 3 clusters.

TF/Easy
Pg:302
kind:f
Ans:True

9.81: An early term for antisocial personality disorder was "moral insanity."

TF/Easy
Pg:303
kind:f
Ans:True

9.82: People with personality disorder frequently do not see themselves as disturbed and so do not seek treatment.

TF/Easy
Pg:305
kind:f
Ans:True

9.83: People with personality disorders usually only meet the criteria for one disorder.

TF/Easy
Pg:305
kind:c
Ans:False

9.84: Temperament is a broader concept than personality.

TF/Easy
Pg:306
kind:f
Ans:False

9.85: A difficult temperament can be adaptive in certain situations.

TF/Easy
Pg:307
kind:f
Ans:True

9.86: Greater consistency in behavior is noted when using global rating scales rather than coding specific behaviors.

TF/Mod
Pg:308
kind:f
Ans:True

9.87: Schizoid personality disorder is characterized by bizarre fantasies and unusual perceptual experiences.

TF/Mod
Pg:310
kind:f
Ans:False

9.88: Persons with schizotypal personality disorder are psychotic and out of touch with reality.

TF/Mod
Pg:310
kind:f
Ans:False

9.89: Only serious criminals meet the criteria for antisocial personality disorder.

TF/Easy
Pg:311
kind:f
Ans:False

9.90: The attention-seeking styles of dress and behavior seen in rock stars are generally considered to be a sign of histrionic personality disorder.

TF/Easy
Pg:313
kind:f
Ans:False

9.91: Obsessive-compulsive disorder is no longer recognized as an anxiety disorder, but is now classified as obsessive-compulsive personality disorder.

TF/Mod
Pg:314
kind:f
Ans:False

9.92: Most personality disorders were not studied extensively until after the publication of DSM-III.

TF/Mod
Pg:316
kind:f
Ans:True

9.93: Most people who meet the criteria for one DSM-IV personality disorder also meet the criteria for another disorder.

TF/Easy
Pg:316
kind:f
Ans:True

9.94: Histrionic personality disorder is more common in women.

TF/Easy
Pg:319
kind:f
Ans:False

9.95: In general, personality disorders are much more common in women than in men.

TF/Easy
Pg:320
kind:f
Ans:False

9.96: According to Moffitt, limited behavioral skills increase the likelihood that a child will continue to show antisocial behaviors into adolescence and adulthood.

TF/Mod
Pg:332
kind:c
Ans:True

9.97: Evaluation of treatment programs for antisocial personality disorder is difficult because of the high rate of alcoholism and substance abuse in this population.

TF/Easy
Pg:333
kind:f
Ans:True

185

Essay Questions

9.98: Describe some of the ways that personality disorders differ from other forms of mental disorder.

Answer: Less impairment; stable rather than episodic course; ego syntonic rather than ego dystonic.

ES Moderate Pages: 302-305 kind: c

9.99: What is the person-situation debate in the study of personality? How has this debate affected methodology and theory?

Answer: Is behavior based on internal personality traits (personality theory), or determined by the specific context in which it occurs (social learning theory)? This debate has engendered better methods for measuring cross-situational consistency (global, aggregate measures). Newer theories endorse an interactional view of situational and personality variables.

ES Moderate Page: 307 kind: c

9.100: Describe the 5-factor model of personality.

Answer: Neuroticism: emotional stability and negative affect.
Extraversion: activity level and interest in people.
Openness to experience: curiosity.
Agreeableness: cooperativeness.
Conscientiousness: persistence and dependability.

ES Moderate Page: 309 kind: c

9.101: The DSM-IV describes personality disorders in terms of discrete categories. Discuss the limitations of this approach.

Answer: Use of discrete categories leaves no way of describing people with traits who don't meet the criteria for a disorder. Because of common overlap in personality disorders, the final diagnosis (either using 1 diagnosis or 2) doesn't provide an accurate description of individual traits. The dimensional approach is more complete, especially for individuals on the boundary of 2 disorders. The dimensional approach is also less complicated, as it is based on 5 dimensions rather than various traits associated with 10 different disorders.

ES Moderate Page: 315 kind: c

9.102: Discuss some of the reasons that some clinicians would believe that histrionic personality disorder is more common in women, even though epidemiological data do not support this conclusion.

Answer: Women may seek treatment more often than men for histrionic personality disorder. Men with histrionic personality disorder may also have substance abuse problems, which are more readily addressed in diagnosis and treatment.

ES   Moderate   Page: 319   kind: c

9.103: Describe how the primate separation model has been used as a tool for understanding the emotional regulation problems seen in borderline personality disorder.

Answer: Young monkeys separated from their mothers and peers experience persistent problems in attachment behavior, negative affect, establishing and maintaining social boundaries, and self-destructive behavior. There may be a similar link between early parental loss or unavailability in humans and borderline personality disorder.

ES   Difficult   Page: 325   kind: c

9.104: Discuss the reasons that psychological treatment of personality disorder is especially difficult.

Answer: Because of the ego syntonic nature of the disorder, patients may show low motivation for or insight about treatment. Personality disorders are rarely present in their "pure" form, and patients may show more than one disorder at a time. The very nature of the disorder makes it difficult to establish a stable, close relationship between the therapist and client.

ES   Difficult   Page: 335   kind: c

Chapter 10
Alcoholism and Substance Use Disorders

Multiple Choice Questions

10.1: DSM-IV defines substance abuse in terms of:　　　　MC/Easy
　　　　　　　　　　　　　　　　　　　　　　　　　　　　Pg:338
　　　a) tolerance and withdrawal　　　　　　　　　　　kind:c
　　　b) craving and lack of control　　　　　　　　　Ans:(d)
　　　c) addiction
　　　d) interference with obligations at work and home

10.2: Polysubstance abuse refers to abuse of:　　　　　MC/Easy
　　　　　　　　　　　　　　　　　　　　　　　　　　　　Pg:338
　　　a) several types of drugs　　　　　　　　　　　　kind:f
　　　b) more serious drugs　　　　　　　　　　　　　Ans:(a)
　　　c) illegal drugs
　　　d) prescription drugs

10.3: A general notion of addition as "excessive　　　MC/Mod
　　　appetite" can apply to many forms of behavior, such　Pg:339
　　　as sex, gambling, and eating. According to this　　kind:c
　　　conceptualization, all of these problem behaviors　Ans:(d)
　　　have in common:

　　　a) moral inferiority
　　　b) neuroticism
　　　c) antisocial tendencies
　　　d) self-destructiveness and diminished control

10.4: A central nervous system depressant that is used to　MC/Mod
　　　relieve anxiety is called:　　　　　　　　　　　Pg:339
　　　　　　　　　　　　　　　　　　　　　　　　　　　　kind:f
　　　a) an hypnotic　　　　　b) an opiate　　　　　　Ans:(d)
　　　c) an analgesic　　　　　d) an anxiolytic

10.5: What type of drug is alcohol?　　　　　　　　　MC/Easy
　　　　　　　　　　　　　　　　　　　　　　　　　　　　Pg:339
　　　a) an opiate　　　　　　　　　　　　　　　　　kind:f
　　　b) an analgesic　　　　　　　　　　　　　　　Ans:(d)
　　　c) a central nervous system stimulant
　　　d) a central nervous system depressant

10.6: Another name for "narcotic analgesic" is:

    a) cannibinoid   b) hypnotic
    c) opiate   d) anxiolytic

MC/Mod
Pg:339
kind:f
Ans:(c)

10.7: Ernest Hemingway suffered from:

    a) cocaine dependence
    b) borderline personality disorder
    c) anxiety disorder
    d) alcohol dependence

MC/Easy
Pg:340
kind:f
Ans:(d)

10.8: Alcohol affects nearly every organ in the body, but an organ that is especially damaged in chronic alcoholism is:

    a) the kidney   b) the liver
    c) the spleen   d) the pancreas

MC/Easy
Pg:340
kind:f
Ans:(b)

10.9: In most states, the current legal limit of alcohol concentration for driving is:

    a) 10 mg alcohol per 100 ml blood
    b) 100 mg alcohol per 100 ml blood
    c) 200 mg alcohol per 100 ml blood
    d) 400 mg alcohol per 100 ml blood

MC/Mod
Pg:342
kind:f
Ans:(b)

10.10: There is an extreme risk of coma leading to toxic death when blood alcohol levels rise above:

    a) 10 mg alcohol per 100 ml blood
    b) 100 mg alcohol per 100 ml blood
    c) 200 mg alcohol per 100 ml blood
    d) 400 mg alcohol per 100 ml blood

MC/Mod
Pg:342
kind:f
Ans:(d)

10.11: Charles is administered a blood alcohol level test and the results show 400 mg alcohol per 100 ml blood. Which of the following characterizes his state?

    a) basically unaffected by the small amount he drank earlier
    b) slightly intoxicated
    c) his driving is probably impaired, but he could walk home
    d) very intoxicated, at risk of slipping into coma

MC/Mod
Pg:342
kind:a
Ans:(d)

10.12: The most useful distinction between people who are dependent on alcohol and those who are not is:

    a) the amount of alcohol consumed each week
    b) legal involvement due to drinking
    c) the number of problems due to drinking
    d) the amount of money spent on alcohol

MC/Mod
Pg:342
kind:c
Ans:(c)

10.13: One example of psychological dependence on alcohol is:

    a) not wanting to drink alone
    b) drinking to control one's emotions
    c) ability to drink more and more over time
    d) cognitive impairments due to alcohol abuse

MC/Mod
Pg:343
kind:c
Ans:(b)

10.14: Tolerance for a psychoactive substance refers to:

    a) psychological dependence
    b) withdrawal
    c) requiring more of a substance to achieve the same effect that lower doses used to achieve
    d) requiring less of a substance to achieve the same effect that higher doses used to achieve

MC/Easy
Pg:344
kind:f
Ans:(c)

10.15: Withdrawal from alcohol occurs because a drinker's biological system:

    a) rebounds after functioning in a chronically depressed state
    b) rebounds after functioning in a chronically stimulated state
    c) is deprived of essential vitamins
    d) has become psychologically dependent

MC/Mod
Pg:344
kind:c
Ans:(a)

10.16: Delirium tremens is the name for:

    a) tolerance for heroine
    b) certain symptoms of withdrawal from alcohol
    c) psychological dependence and craving
    d) Korsakoff's syndrome

MC/Easy
Pg:344
kind:f
Ans:(b)

10.17: A blackout is defined by:

  a) inability to remember what has happened
  b) passing out
  c) dementia
  d) nausea and insomnia

MC/Easy
Pg:345
kind:f
Ans:(a)

10.18: Temperance workers in the 1800s believed that:

  a) alcohol should be legalized
  b) only men should drink alcohol
  c) anyone who drank alcohol would become a
     drunkard
  d) alcohol could be consumed safely in moderation

MC/Mod
Pg:346
kind:c
Ans:(c)

10.19: Temperance workers in the 1800s in the U.S.:

  a) promoted moderate drinking rather than
     drunkenness
  b) believed drinking was acceptable if legal
  c) made a moral argument against drinking
  d) made a scientific argument against drinking

MC/Easy
Pg:346
kind:f
Ans:(c)

10.20: Jellinek, an early researcher on alcoholism,
       believed alcoholism to be a progressive disease.
       By this, he meant that alcoholism:

  a) inevitably got worse and progressed through a
     series of predictable stages
  b) was due to the pressures of modern life
  c) was seen by conservatives as a problem of
     liberals
  d) caused spreading brain deterioration

MC/Mod
Pg:346
kind:c
Ans:(a)

10.21: Based on the responses of members of Alcoholics
       Anonymous in the 1940s and 1950s, Jellinek
       concluded that alcoholism:

  a) can be subdivided into Type 1 and Type 2
  b) follows a predictable and inflexible series of
     4 stages
  c) has a different course depending on the
     individual
  d) is due to chromosomal abnormality

MC/Mod
Pg:346
kind:c
Ans:(b)

10.22: When DSM-I was published in 1952, alcoholism was included under the general heading of:

a) personality disorder
b) adjustment disorder
c) physical conditions related to treatment
d) dementia

MC/Mod
Pg:347
kind:f
Ans:(a)

10.23: In DSM-III, the distinction between substance abuse and substance dependence was created in part because of evidence that:

a) people whose adjustment is impaired by substance use do not all become dependent
b) people who are dependent on substances do not all abuse substances
c) substance abuse is more severe than dependence
d) substance abusers do not suffer serious impairment

MC/Mod
Pg:347
kind:c
Ans:(a)

10.24: In order for a person to be diagnosed with substance dependence in DSM-IV, the person MUST show:

a) tolerance and withdrawal
b) concealed substance use and blackouts
c) delirium tremens
d) a pattern of compulsive use

MC/Mod
Pg:347
kind:c
Ans:(d)

10.25: For research purposes, Cloninger has classified alcoholism into Type 1 and Type 2. The primary conceptual distinction between these two types is the presence or absence of:

a) motivation to stop drinking
b) delirium tremens
c) antisocial traits
d) Korsakoff's psychosis

MC/Diff
Pg:347
kind:c
Ans:(c)

10.26: Cloninger's Type 1 alcoholism, which is found in both men and women, is characterized by:

a) early onset
b) presence of antisocial traits
c) absence of antisocial traits
d) low psychological dependence

MC/Diff
Pg:347
kind:c
Ans:(c)

10.27: Although the course of alcoholism is different in   MC/Mod
       every individual, nearly all cases of alcoholism   Pg:348
       involve: kind:f
                                                                Ans:(c)

       a) onset before age 20
       b) antisocial behavior
       c) alternating periods of heavy use and abstinence
       d) a predictable sequence of phases

10.28: Vaillant's long-term study of patients hospitalized   MC/Mod
       for alcoholism found that on average, patients   Pg:348
       returned for detoxification: kind:f
                                                                Ans:(d)

       a) very rarely
       b) about once every 10 years
       c) about once every 5 years
       d) about twice a year

10.29: One problem which commonly co-occurs with   MC/Easy
       alcoholism is: Pg:349
                                                                kind:f
       a) dependent personality disorder   Ans:(b)
       b) mood disorder
       c) adjustment disorder
       d) schizophrenia

10.30: Some occupations are associated with higher rates   MC/Easy
       of alcoholism, perhaps because they: Pg:349
                                                                kind:c
       a) are degraded by society   Ans:(c)
       b) are male-dominated
       c) lack structured hours
       d) provide low pay

10.31: According to the Epidemiologic Catchment Area (ECA)   MC/Mod
       study, about what percentage of men in the U.S.   Pg:350
       develop problems at some point of their lives due   kind:f
       to prolonged alcohol consumption?   Ans:(c)

       a) 1%   b) 5%
       c) 10%   d) 20%

10.32: After alcohol, the most frequently abused substance   MC/Mod
       is: Pg:350
                                                                kind:f
       a) cocaine   b) cannabis   Ans:(b)
       c) LSD   d) sedatives

10.33: Women are most likely to drink alcohol:　　　　MC/Mod
　　　　　　　　　　　　　　　　　　　　　　　　Pg:351
　　　　a) in old age　　　b) in middle age　　kind:f
　　　　c) as young adults　d) as teenagers　　Ans:(c)

10.34: Gender differences in rates of substance abuse,　MC/Mod
　　　　with men showing more problems than women, are most　Pg:351
　　　　marked in the abuse of:　　　　　　　　kind:f
　　　　　　　　　　　　　　　　　　　　　　　　Ans:(a)
　　　　a) alcohol　　　　　b) marijuana
　　　　c) heroin　　　　　d) cocaine

10.35: Prevalence rates for alcohol dependence are highest　MC/Mod
　　　　among which age group?　　　　　　　　Pg:351
　　　　　　　　　　　　　　　　　　　　　　　　kind:f
　　　　a) adolescents　　　b) young adults　　Ans:(b)
　　　　c) the middle aged　d) the elderly

10.36: Barry and Francesca each weigh 150 pounds. They go　MC/Mod
　　　　out drinking and each has 3 beers. Francesca　Pg:352
　　　　becomes intoxicated sooner, in part because:　kind:a
　　　　　　　　　　　　　　　　　　　　　　　　Ans:(a)
　　　　a) women's bodies have lower water content
　　　　b) men's bodies have lower water content
　　　　c) women's liver functioning is less efficient
　　　　d) men's liver functioning is less efficient

10.37: What is the proportion of drinkers who develop　MC/Mod
　　　　problems?　　　　　　　　　　　　　　Pg:354
　　　　　　　　　　　　　　　　　　　　　　　　kind:f
　　　　a) 1:100　　　　　　b) 1:50　　　　　Ans:(c)
　　　　c) 1:10　　　　　　d) 1:5

10.38: One of the short-term benefits of alcohol　MC/Diff
　　　　consumption that may reinforce further drinking in　Pg:355
　　　　some people is:　　　　　　　　　　　kind:f
　　　　　　　　　　　　　　　　　　　　　　　　Ans:(d)
　　　　a) heightened EEG activity
　　　　b) nystagmus
　　　　c) slowed reaction time
　　　　d) dampened cardiovascular responses to stress

194

10.39: The lifetime prevalence of alcoholism among families of alcoholics is higher than in the general population, by a factor of about:

a) 2
c) 10
b) 3-5
d) 20

10.40: Studies of twins show a moderate influence of genetics in the etiology of alcoholism in males, evident primarily in concordance rates for monozygotic (MZ) twins being much higher than the concordance rates for dizygotic (DZ) twins. Although inconclusive, evidence from studies of alcoholism in female twins suggests that genetics play:

a) no role for women
b) a much greater role for women than for men
c) an equally great role for women and men
d) a slightly smaller role for women than for men

10.41: Studies of the DAUGHTERS of patients with Cloninger's Type 1 and Type 2 alcoholism show increased risk for alcoholism:

a) in both types
c) in Type 2
b) in Type 1
d) in neither type

10.42: Endorphins are most similar pharmacologically to:

a) alcohol
c) morphine
b) cocaine
d) anxiolytics

10.43: Another name for an endorphin is:

a) serotonin
c) endogenous opioid
b) morphine
d) exogenous opioid

10.44: Some scientists believe that alcohol is related to endorphin production based on evidence that:

a) the symptoms of withdrawal from alcohol and heroin are similar
b) the behavioral and pharmacological effects of alcohol and opioids are similar
c) rats given morphine refuse alcohol
d) alcohol is an opioid derivative

10.45: Alcohol produces a depression of the central
nervous system by:

 a) binding directly to receptor sites in the brain
 b) reducing endorphins
 c) decreasing serotonin activity
 d) altering the permeability of neuronal membranes

MC/Diff
Pg:357
kind:f
Ans:(d)

10.46: Cloninger studied rates of alcoholism in children
whose parents showed Type 1 alcoholism (late onset,
non-antisocial traits). He found an increased risk
of alcoholism in children whose adoptive father was
in an unskilled occupation. This increased risk
was thought to be associated with:

 a) low intelligence
 b) poor coping skills
 c) poor nutrition
 d) exposure to heavy recreational drinking

MC/Mod
Pg:358
kind:c
Ans:(d)

10.47: The serotonin hypothesis of alcoholism holds that
intoxication increases the production of serotonin,
correcting a genetic deficiency in serotonin
activity. This can lead to a debilitating process
because when the person sobers up, the serotonin
level:

 a) remains high
 b) drops to levels even below what it was
 c) returns to normal but endorphin levels drop
 d) returns to normal but endorphin levels rise

MC/Mod
Pg:359
kind:c
Ans:(b)

10.48: Traditional learning theory has held that people
drink because:

 a) abstinence is punished through social
    disapproval
 b) parents model drinking behavior and attitudes
 c) drinking occurs on an intermittent
    reinforcement schedule
 d) drinking is reinforced by reductions in fear
    and anxiety

MC/Mod
Pg:360
kind:c
Ans:(d)

10.49: A researcher decides to use a balanced placebo
design rather than a regular placebo design in
order to study the effects of expectations on
subjects' reactions to alcohol consumption. For a
balanced placebo design, the researcher must be
sure to include a condition where subjects:

    a) expect alcohol and get alcohol
    b) expect alcohol and get tonic water
    c) expect tonic water and get alcohol
    d) expect tonic water and get tonic water

MC/Mod
Pg:360
kind:a
Ans:(c)

10.50: A placebo group is typically used in drug studies
to control for:

    a) subjects' expectations about the effects of the
       drug
    b) the effects of high doses
    c) gender differences in drug response
    d) monopolies by big drug companies

MC/Easy
Pg:360
kind:f
Ans:(a)

10.51: The balanced placebo design is a combination of the
placebo and antiplacebo methods. Which of the
following is an example of an antiplacebo condition
in a study of subjects' responses to alcohol?

    a) a person expects to receive alcohol and does
    b) a person expects to receive tonic water and
       does
    c) a person expects to receive tonic water but
       receives alcohol
    d) a person expects to receive alcohol but
       receives tonic water

MC/Diff
Pg:361
kind:c
Ans:(c)

10.52: According to the attention-allocation model, an
intoxicated person shows "alcohol myopia." This
refers to:

    a) wandering eyes when looking up or to the side
    b) self-centeredness
    c) narrowed attention to immediate environmental
       cues
    d) preoccupation with the availability of alcohol

MC/Mod
Pg:362
kind:c
Ans:(c)

10.53: According to the attention-allocation model,   MC/Mod
       consuming alcohol can lead to aggression,   Pg:362
       irresponsible sexual behavior, and drunken excess   kind:c
       because: Ans:(a)

       a) reasoning and inhibition are disrupted
       b) people expect alcohol to have these effects
       c) these behaviors ensure access to more alcohol
       d) intoxicated people want to draw attention to
          themselves

10.54: Isabelle is an anxious person. According to the   MC/Mod
       attention-allocation model, when Isabelle drinks   Pg:362
       alcohol, she might then feel less anxious as long   kind:a
       as she: Ans:(d)

       a) drinks enough to become intoxicated
       b) believes alcohol will relax her
       c) has had relaxing experiences with alcohol in
          the past
       d) is able to distract herself while drinking

10.55: An important element of the classical conditioning   MC/Mod
       model of tolerance is the physiological phenomenon   Pg:363
       called a compensatory response, produced by many   kind:c
       drugs. A compensatory response is: Ans:(b)

       a) a cognitive expectation that the drug will
          affect you
       b) a physiological response that is opposite to
          the drug's effects
       c) a physiological response that mimics the drug's
          effects
       d) a tendency to take more drugs after a period of
          abstinence

10.56: After repeatedly using heroin, a person begins to   MC/Mod
       show an anticipatory reaction to the heroin even   Pg:364
       before it is administered. If he is trying to   kind:a
       reduce his tolerance for heroin by reducing this   Ans:(b)
       anticipatory reaction, he should:

       a) begin to use a different psychoactive substance
       b) take the heroin in a different environmental
          setting
       c) formulate different cognitive expectations
          about heroin's effects
       d) just use heroin in one environment, not in
          several environments

10.57: Detoxification refers to:

MC/Easy
Pg:365
kind:f
Ans:(a)

    a) removal of the drug on which the person is
       dependent
    b) psychotherapy for substance abuse
    c) deterioration of brain tissue secondary to drug
       abuse
    d) symptoms of withdrawal from drug dependence

10.58: The serotonin theory about the etiology of
alcoholism is based in part on evidence that:

MC/Diff
Pg:365
kind:f
Ans:(c)

    a) alcohol and serotonin have opposite chemical
       structures
    b) alcohol and serotonin have the same chemical
       structures
    c) drugs that enhance serotonin transmission can
       decrease alcohol consumption in animals
    d) drugs that enhance serotonin transmission can
       increase alcohol consumption in animals

10.59: Antabuse is a:

MC/Mod
Pg:365
kind:f
Ans:(b)

    a) chemical that enhances the breakdown of alcohol
    b) chemical that blocks the breakdown of alcohol
    c) safe substitute for alcohol
    d) 12-step program for alcoholism

10.60: Larry takes Antabuse and then has a shot of
whiskey. Which is likely to occur?

MC/Easy
Pg:365
kind:a
Ans:(a)

    a) he will become violently ill
    b) he will not feel the effects of the alcohol
    c) he will become intoxicated more quickly
    d) he will become violent

10.61: Alcoholics Anonymous is:

MC/Easy
Pg:366
kind:f
Ans:(a)

    a) a supportive organization based on a spiritual
       approach
    b) a form of treatment based on the medical model
    c) group psychotherapy based on psychodynamic
       principles
    d) group therapy based on humanistic principles

10.62: Alcoholics Anonymous was the first 12-step program.   MC/Easy
As part of recovery, the first step is: Pg:366
                                                             kind:f
a) a recognition that one must recover on one's   Ans:(c)
   own
b) checking into a hospital detox program
c) a spiritual recognition that one is powerless
   over alcohol
d) seeing a psychotherapist

10.63: The 12-step program of Alcoholics Anonymous was   MC/Easy
developed based on: Pg:366
                                                             kind:c
a) spiritual ideas about recovery   Ans:(a)
b) scientific evidence of cognitive changes
   accompanying abstinence
c) biological evidence of changes accompanying
   abstinence
d) psychological theories of defense mechanisms

10.64: One of the most important aspects of Alcoholics   MC/Mod
Anonymous is: Pg:367
                                                             kind:c
a) a stable social network   Ans:(a)
b) biological intervention such as Antabuse
c) emphasis on overall physical health
d) leadership and treatment by a mental health
   professional

10.65: Which of the following characterizes Individualized   MC/Easy
Behavior Therapy for Alcoholics (IBTA), as designed   Pg:367
by Sobell and Sobell?   kind:f
                                                             Ans:(c)
a) use of Antabuse to reduce drinking
b) punishment for drinking
c) training in social skills to resist pressures
   to drink
d) reinforcement for abstinence

10.66: One criticism of Individualized Behavior Therapy
for Alcoholics (IBTA), as designed by Sobell and
Sobell, is that:

    a) there is not enough focus on social skills
    b) there is not enough focus on problem-solving
    c) there is a focus on punishment rather than
       reinforcement
    d) the goal is controlled drinking rather than
       abstinence

MC/Mod
Pg:367
kind:c
Ans:(d)

10.67: The cognitive-behavioral view of relapse prevention
of drug and alcohol dependence places emphasis on
increasing self-efficacy. Self-efficacy is:

    a) a feeling of relaxation
    b) a sense of self-worth
    c) a belief that you can control your own behavior
    d) a realization that you have to recover on your
       own

MC/Mod
Pg:368
kind:c
Ans:(c)

10.68: The cognitive behavioral model of relapse
prevention is concerned with the abstinence
violation effect. This is:

    a) the fact that drinking in public is illegal in
       some states
    b) the pattern of going back to chronic drinking
       if one slips up even a little
    c) a patient's feeling that he or she is being
       controlled by the therapist
    d) a patient's tendency to lie about concealed
       drinking

MC/Mod
Pg:368
kind:c
Ans:(b)

10.69: Rebecca is trying to recover from alcoholism. Her
therapist is trying to help her reduce the
abstinence violation effect. This is a problem for
Rebecca because as soon as she has even a small
drink, she thinks:

    a) "I've messed up; I may as well go ahead and get
       drunk."
    b) "I can recover on my own; I don't need help."
    c) "I am a worthless person."
    d) "I'm only doing something wrong if it's
       illegal."

MC/Mod
Pg:368
kind:a
Ans:(a)

10.70: Which of the following is generally true about treatment for substance abuse and dependence?

   a) evidence shows group therapy is better than individual therapy
   b) long-term outcome depends most on coping and social support
   c) once treatment is finished, relapse is rare
   d) most therapists recommend controlled drinking as a goal

MC/Mod
Pg:368
kind:c
Ans:(b)

True-False Questions

10.71: Substance dependence is more severe than substance abuse.

TF/Easy
Pg:338
kind:f
Ans:True

10.72: Addiction is an older term for substance dependence.

TF/Easy
Pg:338
kind:f
Ans:True

10.73: A chemical substance that alters a person's mood, level of perception, or brain functioning is called a psychoactive substance.

TF/Easy
Pg:339
kind:f
Ans:True

10.74: Nicotine and caffeine are psychoactive substances.

TF/Easy
Pg:339
kind:f
Ans:True

10.75: The DSM-IV employs a different set of criteria to define dependence on different types of psychoactive substances.

TF/Mod
Pg:340
kind:f
Ans:False

10.76: The withdrawal symptoms that follow a cessation in alcohol abuse are usually more pronounced than those following cessation of amphetamine or cocaine abuse.

TF/Mod
Pg:344
kind:f
Ans:True

10.77: The rate of violent crime is actually no higher among men who are dependent on alcohol than it is among men in the general population.

TF/Easy
Pg:345
kind:f
Ans:False

10.78: Drunkenness was not considered to be socially deviant or a symptom of medical illness during Colonial times in America.

TF/Easy
Pg:346
kind:f
Ans:True

10.79: In the DSM-IV, tolerance and withdrawal are required for the diagnosis of substance dependence.

TF/Mod
Pg:347
kind:f
Ans:False

10.80: The difference in drinking patterns seen in men and women in the U.S. is unique to this culture, and is not seen in other countries.

TF/Mod
Pg:351
kind:f
Ans:False

10.81: On average, the age of onset of alcoholism among women is older than it is among men.

TF/Easy
Pg:352
kind:f
Ans:True

10.82: Endorphins are chemicals that are naturally synthesized in the brain.

TF/Easy
Pg:357
kind:f
Ans:True

10.83: The serotonin hypothesis of the etiology of alcoholism assumes that alcohol dependence is caused by a genetically determined overactivity of serotonin.

TF/Diff
Pg:357
kind:f
Ans:False

10.84: Research using a balanced placebo design shows that subjects who believe they ingested alcohol but who actually consumed tonic water show no changes in aggression or sexual behavior.

TF/Mod
Pg:359
kind:f
Ans:False

10.85: Tolerance for psychoactive substances is a biological phenomenon that is unaffected by learning experiences.

TF/Mod
Pg:363
kind:c
Ans:False

10.86: In detoxification from stimulants such as cocaine, administration of the drug can be stopped abruptly.

TF/Easy
Pg:365
kind:f
Ans:True

10.87: Most mental health professional consider controlled drinking to be a realistic goal for people who are dependent on alcohol.

TF/Mod
Pg:367
kind:f
Ans:False

10.88: Most people with substance use disorders are involved in Alcoholics Anonymous or other forms of treatment.

TF/Easy
Pg:368
kind:f
Ans:False

Essay Questions

10.89: Explain why the AMOUNT of alcohol consumed is not the best indicator of an alcohol problem. What are better indicators?

Answer: People vary significantly in the amount of alcohol they can metabolize. This can vary by gender, amount of body fat, physical health, and race. Better indicators are binge drinking and concealed drinking, and the number of social, adjustment, and legal problems that a person encounters related to drinking.

ES   Moderate   Page: 343   kind: c

10.90: Describe Jellinek's disease concept of alcoholism and the 4 phases of the disease's course.

Answer: Jellinek viewed alcoholism as a progressive disorder that invariably got worse over a series of inflexible and predictable stages, which were the same for everyone. The prealcoholic phase is characterized by social drinking and drinking to relieve tension. The prodromal phase is characterized by concealed drinking and blackouts. The crucial phase is characterized by daytime drinking and impairment in social and occupational functioning and judgment. The chronic phase is characterized by the person living to drink, and experiencing withdrawal if not drinking.

ES   Moderate   Pages: 346-347   kind: c

10.91: Discuss the methodological problems that make it difficult to collect epidemiological information on substance abuse and substance dependence.

Answer: Research over the years has lacked a consistent definition of substance abuse and substance dependence. The problems associated with these problems show great variability across the lifespan. These problems often co-occur with other psychiatric problems, making research conclusions difficult. Finally, because many psychoactive drugs are illegal, it is difficult to get accurate reports about people's drug use.

   ES   Moderate   Pages: 349-350   kind: c

10.92: Describe some of the issues involved in substance dependence among the elderly.

Answer: The elderly show the lowest rates of alcoholism, and rarely use illegal drugs. However, they show problems with prescription drugs, partly because they are often prescribed several drugs at once, and they show increased sensitivity to drug toxicity. Their withdrawal from substances can be more prolonged and more severe than in younger persons. Occupational and social impairment may be less noticeable, however, because the elderly are no longer working and may not be living with their own family.

   ES   Moderate   Pages: 351-352   kind: c

10.93: Discuss the ways that parent behaviors influence the likelihood that an adolescent will abuse substances.

Answer: Parents might model the use of substances for recreational or stress-reduction purposes. Adolescents might be influenced by their parents' positive attitudes and expectations about the effects of substance use. If the parents are alcoholic, they may not provide sufficient monitoring of the adolescent. If the parents show high conflict and negative affect, the adolescent may be motivated to spend more time with peers.

   ES   Moderate   Pages: 354-355   kind: c

10.94: Review the evidence for the serotonin model of alcoholism.

Answer: Animals reared to show a high or low preference for alcohol have different levels of brain serotonin. Similarly, different patterns of alcoholism in humans (early onset with family history vs. late onset without family history) show different serotonin levels. Serotonin Reuptake Inhibitors enhance serotonin transmission and decrease voluntary alcohol consumption in humans.

ES Moderate Page: 359 kind: c

10.95: Explain the classical conditioning model of tolerance and withdrawal.

Answer: This model combines biological phenomena with learning processes. Many drugs produce a compensatory response--i.e., the body reacts in a manner that is opposite the drug effects. Through repeated use, the body begins to show the compensatory effects in anticipation of drug administration. Tolerance may develop when this anticipatory reaction is strengthened through association with environmental cues, and leads to further drug use. Withdrawal may be viewed as the presence of compensatory effects in the absence of drug use.

ES Difficult Pages: 363-364 kind: c

Chapter 11
Sexual and Gender Identity Disorders

Multiple Choice Questions

11.1: Which of the following is characteristic of a man with a paraphilia?

    a) shows aversion to his own sexuality
    b) is sexually aroused by unusual situations or objects
    c) is physically incapable of having an erection
    d) shows inhibited sex drive and low arousal

MC/Easy
Pg:374
kind:f
Ans:(b)

11.2: William Masters and Virginia Johnson are best known for:

    a) documenting the diversity of normal sexual behavior
    b) describing the human sexual response cycle
    c) writing about childhood sexuality
    d) classifying the perversions

MC/Mod
Pg:374
kind:c
Ans:(b)

11.3: Masters and Johnson were able to describe the human sexual response cycle based on:

    a) observations of human couples having intercourse
    b) analogue studies of the sexual behavior of primates
    c) detailed interviews with thousands of adults
    d) cross-cultural analysis of texts on human sexuality

MC/Mod
Pg:374
kind:f
Ans:(a)

11.4: Some of the most dramatic physiological changes during sexual excitement are due to vasocongestion. This refers to increases in:

    a) respiration rates
    b) muscular tension
    c) neurotransmitter activity
    d) engorgement of blood vessels

MC/Easy
Pg:375
kind:f
Ans:(d)

11.5: Jonah has just reached orgasm and find that he is
unable to get an erection again. Although this
greatly concerns him, it is actually a normal
phenomenon known as:

MC/Mod
Pg:376
kind:a
Ans:(a)

a) the refractory period
b) vasocongestion
c) plateau
d) dyspareunia

11.6: The final phase of the human sexual response cycle
is:

MC/Easy
Pg:376
kind:f
Ans:(c)

a) orgasm   b) plateau
c) resolution   d) vasocongestion

11.7: In the 18th and 19th century, masturbation was
considered to be:

MC/Easy
Pg:377
kind:f
Ans:(a)

a) the cause of physical and mental disorders
b) a natural part of sexuality
c) a sign of possession and witchcraft
d) an important part of hygiene

11.8: With respect to sexuality, medical authorities in
the 18th and 19th centuries were most concerned
about:

MC/Mod
Pg:377
kind:f
Ans:(b)

a) subjective dissatisfaction
b) excessive sexual activity
c) impaired sexual performance
d) inhibited sex drive

11.9: Krafft-Ebing's classification of "sexual neuroses,"
proposed at the beginning of the 20th century,
focused primarily on:

MC/Mod
Pg:377
kind:f
Ans:(a)

a) perversions   b) erectile impairment
c) ejaculatory control d) inhibited sex drive

11.10: Havelock Ellis, the author of a series of influential monographs on the psychology of sexual behavior, made an important impact at the turn of the century because he:

MC/Mod
Pg:378
kind:c
Ans:(d)

a) argued against Freud's notion of children as sexual beings
b) listed a limited number of sexual behaviors as "normal"
c) classified the perversions as "sexual neuroses"
d) saw masturbation and homosexuality as normal

11.11: Who was the biologist who, through interviews with thousands of men and women in the 1930s and 1940s, obtained scientific evidence about the diversity of normal sexual behavior?

MC/Mod
Pg:378
kind:f
Ans:(a)

a) Alfred Kinsey
b) Havelock Ellis
c) Richard von Krafft-Ebing
d) William Masters

11.12: Which of the following was characteristic of the interviews Kinsey conducted in the 1930s and 1940s about sexual behavior?

MC/Mod
Pg:378
kind:c
Ans:(d)

a) they focused primarily on subjective distress
b) they classified perversions as sadism, masochism, and fetishism
c) they were structured to make psychiatric diagnosis possible
d) they focused on experiences that resulted in orgasm

11.13: Based on interviews with 18,000 men and women in the 1930s and 1940s, Kinsey concluded that:

MC/Mod
Pg:378
kind:c
Ans:(b)

a) homosexuality was a perversion
b) distinctions between sexual orientations were essentially meaningless
c) low sexual desire is a form of psychopathology
d) there is little diversity in normal sexual behaviors

11.14: The early descriptions of sexual disorders in the DSM-I were most influenced by:

    a) Kinsey's views on biology
    b) Masters and Johnson's laboratory data
    c) Ellis' monographs on sexuality
    d) psychodynamic theory

MC/Mod
Pg:378
kind:c
Ans:(d)

11.15: In the past, sexual deviations were considered to be a form of:

    a) anxiety disorder
    b) mood disorder
    c) schizophrenia
    d) personality disorder

MC/Mod
Pg:378
kind:f
Ans:(d)

11.16: Homosexuality was eventually removed from the DSM's list of mental illnesses. The most immediate precipitant of this change was:

    a) the influence of psychodynamic therapists
    b) scientific evidence regarding the prevalence of homosexuality
    c) political pressure from gay rights groups
    d) several APA board members identifying themselves as gay

MC/Mod
Pg:379
kind:f
Ans:(c)

11.17: As the American Psychiatric Association began to reconsider whether homosexuality should be removed as a diagnostic category, they began to change their definition of what constituted a mental disorder. Specifically, they decided that in order to be considered a mental disorder, a condition should:

    a) be experienced as uncontrollable, not as a choice
    b) be statistically rare
    c) involve personal distress or social impairment
    d) be viewed as a problem in any culture

MC/Mod
Pg:379
kind:c
Ans:(c)

11.18: In the DSM-III, increased emphasis was placed on   MC/Mod
sexual dysfunction. Specific types of sexual   Pg:379
dysfunction were listed in terms of: kind:c
                                                                  Ans:(c)

    a) associated personality disorders
    b) sexual orientation and interests
    c) interruptions in the response cycle
    d) psychoanalytic notions of ego development

11.19: Hypoactive sexual desire refers to: MC/Easy
                                                                  Pg:381
    a) excessive sex drive   kind:f
    b) sexual attraction to unusual objects   Ans:(d)
    c) situational sexual dysfunction
    d) low sex drive

11.20: When erectile dysfunction occurs, a man: MC/Mod
                                                                  Pg:382
    a) is not erect because he is not subjectively   kind:f
       aroused   Ans:(b)
    b) may be subjectively aroused but blood does not
       flow to his penis
    c) ejaculates immediately upon insertion during
       intercourse
    d) is by definition experiencing dyspareunia

11.21: Inhibited sexual arousal in women is characterized   MC/Mod
by sexual desire that is not accompanied by   Pg:382
physiological responses necessary to achieve   kind:c
intercourse. In this respect, inhibited sexual   Ans:(b)
arousal is most similar to which disorder in men?

    a) premature ejaculation
    b) erectile dysfunction
    c) hypoactive sexual dysfunction
    d) dyspareunia

11.22: Sexual arousal is considered by psychologists to be   MC/Mod
a hypothetical construct because: Pg:383
                                                                  kind:c
    a) it can be objectively measured for research   Ans:(d)
       purposes
    b) it has such diverse expression across
       individuals
    c) its definition differs across cultures
    d) it cannot be measured directly

11.23: An operational definition is based on:

    a) measurable characteristics of a phenomenon
    b) theoretical ideas, not observable data
    c) conventional ideas, not scientific measurement
    d) treatment guidelines for psychiatric disorders

MC/Mod
Pg:383
kind:c
Ans:(a)

11.24: What does a penile plethysmograph do?

    a) allows a man to obtain an artificial erection
    b) helps a man to delay ejaculation
    c) measures changes in the circumference of the penis
    d) measures time taken to reach orgasm

MC/Mod
Pg:383
kind:f
Ans:(c)

11.25: What does a vaginal photometer measure?

    a) lubrication due to sexual arousal
    b) blood flow to the walls of the vagina
    c) rhythmicity of vaginal contractions
    d) time taken to reach orgasm

MC/Mod
Pg:383
kind:f
Ans:(b)

11.26: Dyspareunia refers to:

    a) sexual attraction to unusual objects
    b) premature ejaculation
    c) sexual aversion
    d) genital pain associated with sexual activity

MC/Mod
Pg:384
kind:f
Ans:(d)

11.27: Which of the following characterizes a woman whose orgasmic impairment is generalized?

    a) she has never achieved orgasm by any means
    b) she can reach orgasm only through masturbation
    c) she is averse to all forms of sexual expression
    d) she can reach orgasm with her lover, but not with her husband

MC/Mod
Pg:384
kind:c
Ans:(a)

11.28: Which of the following is true about the epidemiology of dyspareunia?

    a) it occurs only in women
    b) it is considered to be much more common in women
    c) it occurs only in men
    d) it is considered to be much more common in men

MC/Easy
Pg:384
kind:f
Ans:(b)

11.29: Vaginismus is:

    a) a viral infection caused by a sexually
       transmitted disease
    b) a pseudohermaphroditic condition
    c) involuntary muscle spasms that interfere with
       intercourse
    d) a male's desire to be female

MC/Mod
Pg:385
kind:f
Ans:(c)

11.30: Muriel has vaginismus. Besides difficulty having
intercourse, she is likely to have difficulty:

    a) masturbating to orgasm
    b) being sexually responsive in any way
    c) using tampons or getting a vaginal examination
    d) being sexually aroused by men

MC/Mod
Pg:385
kind:a
Ans:(c)

11.31: Research on people's complaints about their sexual
relationships show that among happily married
couples, both men and women report most
dissatisfaction resulting from:

    a) emotional factors rather than physiological
       factors
    b) problems that interfere with arousal
    c) problems that interfere with orgasm
    d) individual problems rather than relationship
       problems

MC/Diff
Pg:386
kind:c
Ans:(a)

11.32: As women get older, one change in their
physiological response to erotic stimuli is:

    a) slower rate of lubrication
    b) less responsiveness in the clitoris
    c) increased risk of vaginismus
    d) increased blood flow to the vaginal walls

MC/Easy
Pg:387
kind:f
Ans:(a)

11.33: Which of the following describes the sexual
performance of elderly men?

    a) very few men this age obtain an erection
    b) over half of elderly men have no trouble
       obtaining an erection
    c) sex drive and erectile functioning remain
       essentially unchanged
    d) erection is rarely a problem, but premature
       ejaculation usually is

MC/Mod
Pg:387
kind:f
Ans:(b)

11.34: Which of the following characterizes the effect of
very low levels of testosterone in males?

    a) lack of erection when viewing erotica
    b) attraction to homosexual stimuli
    c) erectile dysfunction
    d) inhibited response to sexual fantasies

MC/Mod
Pg:388
kind:f
Ans:(d)

11.35: Which of the following characterizes the
association between testosterone levels and men's
sexual appetite or level of desire?

    a) there is no association
    b) there is a nearly 1:1 ratio between
       testosterone levels and desire
    c) very high levels of testosterone predict
       excessive interest
    d) very low levels of testosterone predict
       inhibited desire

MC/Mod
Pg:388
kind:f
Ans:(d)

11.36: Which of the following is a common physical cause
of erectile dysfunction?

    a) liver cirrhosis   b) diabetes
    c) sickle cell anemia   d) Grave's disease

MC/Easy
Pg:388
kind:f
Ans:(b)

11.37: Which tends to be true of the psychological
experiences of men with erectile disorder?

    a) unpleasant emotions when aroused in the
       presence of erotic stimuli
    b) disgust related to most forms of sexual
       expression
    c) excessive interest in erotica
    d) arousal in response to stimuli outside of
       personal relationships

MC/Easy
Pg:389
kind:f
Ans:(a)

11.38: Alfred Kinsey, a biologist who studied human sexuality, concluded that from an evolutionary viewpoint, premature ejaculation:

    a) allows the male fewer opportunities for intercourse
    b) reduces the amount of time the female is protected by the male from predators
    c) is not a form of dysfunction from a biological perspective
    d) reduces the female's chances of pregnancy and reproduction

MC/Mod
Pg:389
kind:c
Ans:(c)

11.39: Compared to women born in earlier decades, women born in more recent decades:

    a) are more likely to reach orgasm
    b) complain less often about vaginismus
    c) show higher rates of paraphilias
    d) rarely complain of dyspareunia

MC/Easy
Pg:390
kind:f
Ans:(a)

11.40: Compared to women who have regular orgasms, women who do not have regular orgasms:

    a) feel more guilty about sex
    b) are less aroused when watching explicitly sexual films
    c) are less sure of their sexual orientation
    d) have less sensate focus

MC/Mod
Pg:390
kind:c
Ans:(a)

11.41: Who was (or were) known for pioneering work in developing a short-term, skills-oriented system for treating sexual dysfunction?

    a) Masters and Johnson   b) Ellis
    c) Kinsey   d) Hite

MC/Easy
Pg:390
kind:f
Ans:(a)

11.42: One change in sex therapy over the last 25 years has been less focus on:

    a) the use of medication
    b) desire disorders
    c) intrapsychic conflicts
    d) family systems

MC/Mod
Pg:390
kind:c
Ans:(c)

11.43: Sensate focus is a cornerstone of sex therapy as developed by Masters and Johnson. The rationale for sensate focus is the need for the couple to:

 a) rule out medical or physical causes of sexual dysfunction
 b) understand intrapsychic conflicts
 c) get support from other couples with similar problems
 d) enjoy the physical pleasure of touching

MC/Mod
Pg:391
kind:c
Ans:(d)

11.44: Maria and John go to a therapist because they consistently have difficulty accomplishing intercourse. The therapist recommends a procedure called sensate focus. If Maria and John follow through with this recommendation, which of the following are they likely to do next?

 a) explore their painful emotions in therapy
 b) go to a physician, to rule out medical problems
 c) spend time together relaxing and holding hands
 d) attempt to have intercourse every night for a week

MC/Mod
Pg:391
kind:a
Ans:(c)

11.45: The success of sensate focus in therapy to overcome sexual dysfunction depends to a large extent on scheduling. Specifically, it is important that the couple:

 a) have similar expectations about the frequency of sex
 b) establish a corresponding rhythm during intercourse
 c) engage in intercourse at different times of the day
 d) set aside quiet time and a private place for sex

MC/Mod
Pg:391
kind:c
Ans:(d)

11.46: Some gay men who dress as women refer to themselves as "drag queens." This behavior is not considered to be a transvestic fetish because for drag queens, cross-dressing:

 a) is not illegal
 b) is only done periodically
 c) is a compulsion
 d) is not associated with sexual arousal

MC/Mod
Pg:392
kind:f
Ans:(d)

216

11.47: Carlos often fantasizes about walking past his   MC/Mod
       window in the nude, so that his female neighbors   Pg:392
       will see him. Although the fantasy is   kind:a
       exhibitionistic, this would not be classified as a   Ans:(d)
       paraphilia because:

       a) the fantasy involves people, not objects
       b) this is not an unusual urge
       c) he does not need the fantasy to become aroused
       d) he has not acted on the urge

11.48: The central problem in paraphilias is that: MC/Mod
                                                                           Pg:393
       a) sexual desire is inhibited   kind:c
       b) a physiological problem prevents arousal   Ans:(c)
       c) sexual arousal is detached from a caring adult
          relationship
       d) the individual feels no guilt about the
          behavior

11.49: Paraphilias have been compared to addictions   MC/Mod
       because both these problems involve: Pg:393
                                                                           kind:c
       a) a genetic predisposition   Ans:(d)
       b) illegal activity
       c) a lack of guilt
       d) a feeling of compulsion

11.50: Men with paraphilias have often been noted to be: MC/Mod
                                                                           Pg:394
       a) homosexual   kind:c
       b) lacking in guilt   Ans:(c)
       c) timid and of low self-esteem
       d) addicted to substances

11.51: A conservative estimate of rape prevalence, based   MC/Mod
       on a national survey conducted by the National   Pg:394
       Victims Center, is that what percentage of adult   kind:f
       women in the U.S. have been raped?   Ans:(c)

       a) 1%   b) 5%
       c) 14%   d) 32%

11.52: Charles finds it impossible to reach orgasm without
holding or looking at a woman's shoe. This problem
is a type of paraphilia known as:

    a) frotteurism
    b) fetishism
    c) transvestic fetishism
    d) crossing

MC/Mod
Pg:394
kind:a
Ans:(b)

11.53: A person with a paraphilia known as frotteurism
would be likely to do which of the following?

    a) feel a need to see a certain object to reach
       orgasm
    b) rub up against someone in a crowded subway
    c) expose himself to his neighbors
    d) feel aroused when he is hit or kicked

MC/Mod
Pg:394
kind:a
Ans:(b)

11.54: Sexual sadism involves sexual arousal associated
with:

    a) feeling pain and humiliation
    b) exposing oneself
    c) rubbing up against someone
    d) hurting or humiliating someone else

MC/Easy
Pg:394
kind:f
Ans:(d)

11.55: Rape was not included as a paraphilia in DSM-IV
because:

    a) the focus of the sex drive is not an inanimate
       object
    b) rape is often not sexually motivated
    c) rape is too common a problem to be considered a
       paraphilia
    d) rape is a legal, not psychological problem

MC/Mod
Pg:394
kind:c
Ans:(b)

11.56: Knight and Prentky identified 4 subtypes of
convicted rapists. According to this
classification scheme, what category would describe
a man who is preoccupied with nonviolent sexual
fantasies, shows deficits in his ability to process
social cues from women, and has feelings of
inferiority?

    a) vindictive   b) opportunistic
    c) nonsadistic   d) sadistic

MC/Mod
Pg:395
kind:c
Ans:(c)

11.57: Knight and Prentky classify convicted rapists as sexually and nonsexually motivated. Research evidence that supports the validity of this distinction indicates that convicted rapists who are classified as sexually motivated:

a) show other paraphilias
b) show erectile difficulty if not fantasizing about rape
c) are more likely to have been sexually abused as children
d) show more sexual arousal when listening to rape scenes

MC/Mod
Pg:395
kind:c
Ans:(d)

11.58: "Crossing" of paraphilic behaviors refers to the fact that:

a) these behaviors are against cultural norms
b) people with these problems are unsure of their sexual orientation
c) almost all paraphiliacs cross-dress
d) people who exhibit one paraphilia often exhibit others

MC/Easy
Pg:396
kind:f
Ans:(d)

11.59: Studies of convicted rapists must be interpreted with caution. One reason for this is that, of rapes that are reported to the police, the proportion that end up in conviction is only around:

a) 5%   b) 10%
c) 25%   d) 50%

MC/Diff
Pg:396
kind:f
Ans:(b)

11.60: Most paraphilias are almost always exhibited by men, with the exception of:

a) frotteurism   b) exhibitionism
c) masochism   d) fetishism

MC/Diff
Pg:396
kind:f
Ans:(c)

11.61: Sexual masochism is:

a) equally likely in men and women
b) slightly more likely in men than in women
c) slightly more likely in women than in men
d) almost always shown only by men

MC/Mod
Pg:396
kind:f
Ans:(a)

11.62: Glenn Wilson, a British ethologist, has explained   MC/Mod
the development of fetishes in terms of prepared   Pg:397
learning. According to this view, males are   kind:c
programmed to respond sexually to: Ans:(b)

a) partners who increase the likelihood of
reproduction
b) visual, not emotional, stimuli
c) features that are opposite to those of their
mother
d) sensations they experience during breast
feeding

11.63: A person with a paraphilia is likely to show: MC/Mod
Pg:398
a) normal heterosexual relationships   kind:c
b) limited intimacy with other adults   Ans:(b)
c) confusion about gender identity
d) an outgoing personality

11.64: According to John Money, a person's "lovemap," a   MC/Mod
mental picture representing a person's ideal sexual   Pg:398
relationship, can become distorted if a man: kind:c
Ans:(c)
a) does not associate sexual arousal with parts of
the mother's body
b) did not have an opposite-sex parental figure
c) cannot integrate romantic attachment and sexual
desire
d) misses a critical phase in which sexual stimuli
are "imprinted"

11.65: Extensive interviews with people who are most   MC/Diff
involved in sexual sadism and masochism have led   Pg:399
researchers to hypothesize that, as children, these   kind:c
people: Ans:(a)

a) used sexual fantasy to counter extreme pain
b) experienced little sexual arousal
c) experienced little physical pain
d) had underaroused biological systems

220

11.66: One biological perspective on the etiology of sexual sadism and masochism concerns:

a) inhibited excitatory systems
b) diminished pain sensitivity
c) unusual patterns of vasocongestion
d) conditioned release of endorphins

MC/Mod
Pg:399
kind:c
Ans:(d)

11.67: Men with paraphilias usually enter treatment:

a) voluntarily
b) by referral from the legal systems
c) for substance abuse problems, not sexual problems
d) by referral from marital therapists

MC/Easy
Pg:399
kind:f
Ans:(b)

11.68: Michael is ordered to undergo aversion therapy for pedophilia. Which of the following is an example of what this treatment might entail?

a) therapy to increase insight to the consequences of pedophilia
b) confrontation by other men with similar problems
c) education about sexual norms
d) receiving electrical shock when sexually aroused by pictures of children

MC/Mod
Pg:399
kind:a
Ans:(d)

11.69: Gender identity is usually fixed by what age?

a) at birth   b) at age 1
c) at age 2-3   d) at age 10

MC/Easy
Pg:400
kind:f
Ans:(c)

11.70: Which of the following statements is an expression of gender identity?

a) "I have a penis."
b) "I like to wrestle and play GI Joe."
c) "I'm a boy."
d) "I'm heterosexual."

MC/Mod
Pg:400
kind:a
Ans:(c)

11.71: Another name for severe gender identity disorder in adults is:

    a) transvestic fetishism
    b) transsexualism
    c) homosexuality
    d) pseudohermaphroditism

MC/Mod
Pg:401
kind:f
Ans:(b)

11.72: Which of the following characterizes a man with gender identity disorder?

    a) a delusional belief that he is a woman
    b) sexually aroused by dressing as a woman
    c) has male and female sex organs
    d) believes that in spite of his anatomy, he is more like a woman

MC/Mod
Pg:401
kind:c
Ans:(d)

11.73: Which of the following is characterized by sexual arousal when dressing in clothing of the opposite gender?

    a) gender identity disorder
    b) transsexuality
    c) transvestic fetishism
    d) pseudohermaphroditism

MC/Mod
Pg:401
kind:c
Ans:(c)

11.74: Children with pseudohermaphroditic conditions are genetically male but don't show male physical characteristics until they reach adolescence. These children are usually raised as girls. At adolescence, they:

    a) develop gender identity disorder
    b) easily adopt a male gender identity
    c) view themselves as homosexual
    d) have no sexual interest

MC/Mod
Pg:402
kind:c
Ans:(b)

11.75: The ease with which pseudohermaphrodites adopt a male gender identity at adolescence seems to suggest that:

    a) learning can override hormonal influences
    b) secondary sex characteristics determine gender identity
    c) social reinforcement and norms dictate gender identity
    d) prenatal hormones affect later gender identity

MC/Mod
Pg:402
kind:c
Ans:(d)

11.76: One of the documented benefits of sex reassignment surgery is:

    a) increased sex drive
    b) reduced anxiety and depression
    c) improved sensate focus
    d) decreased transvestic fetishism

MC/Mod
Pg:402
kind:c
Ans:(b)

True-False Questions

11.77: Inhibited sexual desire can be considered a sexual dysfunction if it causes the person distress.

TF/Easy
Pg:374
kind:f
Ans:True

11.78: Inhibited sexual desire is considered a paraphilia.

TF/Easy
Pg:374
kind:f
Ans:False

11.79: Men and women show the same sequence of phases in the sexual response cycle.

TF/Easy
Pg:374
kind:f
Ans:True

11.80: Kinsey found that it is common for men and women who consider themselves to be heterosexual to have homosexual fantasies and experiences.

TF/Mod
Pg:378
kind:f
Ans:True

11.81: According to DSM-I and DSM-II, homosexuality was by definition a form of mental disorder.

TF/Easy
Pg:378
kind:f
Ans:True

11.82: Sylvia takes a prescription drug that causes decreased sensation in her pelvic area. According to the DSM-IV, she would be diagnosed with a sexual disorder if this caused her distress.

TF/Mod
Pg:380
kind:a
Ans:False

11.83: Sexual aversion disorder is associated with less anxiety and fear than is hypoactive sexual disorder.

TF/Easy
Pg:381
kind:c
Ans:False

11.84: In normal women, there is a nearly 1:1 correspondence between subjective sexual arousal and physiological measures such as vaginal lubrication or vasocongestion.

TF/Mod
Pg:382
kind:f
Ans:False

11.85: Studies of people living in various communities show that people report more sexual dysfunction when responding to a questionnaire than when interviewed.

TF/Mod
Pg:386
kind:f
Ans:False

11.86: People with depressive disorders often experience decreased sexual desire.

TF/Easy
Pg:388
kind:f
Ans:True

11.87: Sexually dysfunctional men are more likely than sexually nondysfunctional men to have mistaken beliefs about human sexuality.

TF/Easy
Pg:389
kind:f
Ans:True

11.88: In order to be diagnosed with a paraphilia, the individual must also show a sexual dysfunction involving desire, arousal, or orgasm during conventional sexual behavior with a partner.

TF/Mod
Pg:392
kind:c
Ans:False

11.89: Frotteurism is a type of paraphilia that is characterized by sexually rubbing up against someone without consent.

TF/Easy
Pg:394
kind:f
Ans:True

11.90: By definition, sexual masochism involves arousal associated with simulated fantasy play where the other person pretends to inflict pain.

TF/Mod
Pg:394
kind:c
Ans:False

11.91: Rape is considered to be a type of paraphilia according to the DSM-IV.

TF/Mod
Pg:394
kind:f
Ans:False

11.92: Research indicates that rape is motivated by both aggressive and sexual components, in various mixtures.

TF/Mod
Pg:395
kind:c
Ans:True

11.93: Most people with paraphilias enter treatment on a voluntary basis.

TF/Easy
Pg:399
kind:f
Ans:False

11.94: Behavioral programs focusing on social skills are thought to be more effective than aversion therapy in the treatment of paraphilias.

TF/Mod
Pg:399
kind:c
Ans:True

11.95: Another term for "transvestite" is "transsexual."

TF/Mod
Pg:401
kind:f
Ans:False

11.96: Among people who present for treatment, it is more common for women to express gender identity disorder than it is for men.

TF/Mod
Pg:401
kind:f
Ans:False

11.97: Patients who request sex reassignment surgery have a disorder known as transsexualism.

TF/Mod
Pg:402
kind:f
Ans:True

Essay Questions

11.98: Describe Freud's contributions to the understanding of human sexuality.

Answer: Freud addressed the issues of children's sexuality and sexual conflict within the family. He held that sexual impulses were a primary motivator for behavior, and that psychological problems can result from trying to deny or repress one's sexuality.

ES   Moderate   Page: 378   kind: c

11.99: The penile plethysmograph and the vaginal photometer measure physiological events directly related to sexual arousal, but they do not measure sexual arousal itself. Instead, they are said to be reflections of a hypothetical construct called "sexual arousal." Using this example, explain the following terms: hypothetical construct, construct validity, and operational definition.

Answer: A hypothetical construct is a theoretical idea that refers to something that can't be observed directly. For example, arousal involves a subjective feeling of being aroused, which cannot be directly observed. In order to use such an idea scientifically, it must be defined in terms of observable indicators, even if these indicators do not define the idea completely. These observable indicators are the operational definition. In the case of arousal, observable factors such as penile circumference and vaginal engorgement are used as indicators of arousal. If these indicators turn out to be related to other indicators of arousal, such as the person's subjective report, then the indicators are said to have construct validity. This means that they are thought to be valid, if incomplete, indicators of the hypothetical construct.

ES   Difficult   Page: 383   kind: c

11.100: Explain why some paraphilias are considered by ethologists to be "courtship disorders."

Answer: Primate sexual behavior involves three stages: location and appraisal of potential partners; exchange of signals of mutual interest; and tactile interactions that set the stage for intercourse. The paraphilias of voyeurism, exhibitionism, and frotteurism in humans may be aberrations of these basic behaviors.

ES   Moderate   Pages: 397-398   kind: c

11.101: Explain what cases of pseudohermaphroditism tell us about what factors influence the development of gender identity.

Answer: Pseudohermaphrodites are genetically male but are born with ambiguous genitalia. Prenatally, they are exposed to male hormones, but the effects of these hormones are not apparent until adolescence, when the individual begins to show male sex characteristics. Many of these people are raised as girls, but then make an easy transition to a male gender identity at adolescence. This suggests that prenatal sex hormones, rather than how the person is raised or socialized, determine later gender identity.

ES   Moderate   Pages: 401-402   kind: c

Chapter 12
Schizophrenic Disorders

Multiple Choice Questions

12.1: Which of the following is true about the symptoms
of schizophrenia?

   a) all schizophrenics have at least one core
      symptom in common
   b) psychosis is not found in any condition other
      than schizophrenia
   c) "negative" symptoms indicate the absence of
      schizophrenia
   d) drug-induced psychosis is not considered
      schizophrenic

MC/Diff
Pg:406
kind:c
Ans:(d)

12.2: Which of the following is an example of a negative
symptom of schizophrenia?

   a) hallucination   b) social withdrawal
   c) delusions   d) disorganized speech

MC/Mod
Pg:406
kind:c
Ans:(b)

12.3: Which of the following is an example of a positive
symptom of schizophrenia?

   a) hallucination   b) social withdrawal
   c) lack of initiative d) flat affect

MC/Mod
Pg:406
kind:c
Ans:(a)

12.4: "Negative" symptoms of schizophrenia are
characterized by:

   a) a negative attitude
   b) signs of recovery
   c) hallucinations and delusions
   d) an absence of normal functioning

MC/Mod
Pg:406
kind:c
Ans:(d)

12.5: The prodromal phase of schizophrenia occurs:

   a) at the point of greatest disturbance
   b) following the active phase
   c) when the patient is treated with neuroleptic
      medications
   d) before active psychotic symptoms are present

MC/Mod
Pg:407
kind:f
Ans:(d)

12.6: In January Rita is beginning to perform poorly at work, is neglecting her appearance, is becoming withdrawn, and is showing some odd behaviors. In March she shows the full-blown symptoms of schizophrenia. Her behavior in January can be considered part of which phase of the disorder?

MC/Mod
Pg:407
kind:a
Ans:(d)

a) active
b) residual
c) undifferentiated
d) prodromal

12.7: Schizophreniform disorder is distinguished from schizophrenic disorder in that schizophreniform disorder is characterized by:

MC/Mod
Pg:409
kind:c
Ans:(d)

a) lack of psychotic symptoms
b) more severe psychotic symptoms
c) longer duration of psychotic symptoms
d) shorter duration of psychotic symptoms

12.8: An hallucination as experienced by a schizophrenic patient:

MC/Mod
Pg:410
kind:c
Ans:(a)

a) seems to the patient to be perfectly real
b) is always frightening to the patient
c) usually occurs once and then goes away
d) seems to the patient to be a trick of his or her imagination

12.9: Which of the following is true about the association between delusions and hallucinations?

MC/Mod
Pg:410
kind:c
Ans:(a)

a) delusions may develop from attempts to understand hallucinations
b) delusions may be so stressful that the patient hallucinates
c) patients usually show either delusions or hallucinations, not both
d) drugs used to treat hallucinations often intensify delusions

12.10: Delusions are:

MC/Easy
Pg:410
kind:f
Ans:(a)

a) rigidly held, idiosyncratic beliefs
b) sensory experiences in the absence of external stimuli
c) examples of disorganized speech
d) lifelong convictions, sometimes held by one's cultural group

228

12.11: Disorganized speech has also been known as:

    a) delusion   b) tardive dyskinesia
    c) catatonia   d) thought disorder

MC/Easy
Pg:411
kind:f
Ans:(d)

12.12: Disorganized speech is characterized by:

    a) poorly communicated meaning
    b) lack of grammatical structure
    c) poor articulation
    d) strong convictions about preposterous ideas

MC/Mod
Pg:411
kind:c
Ans:(a)

12.13: During an interview, a schizophrenic patient gives answers that seem at first to be in response to the question, but which then get lost in irrelevant details. This phenomenon is known as:

    a) hallucination   b) tangentiality
    c) perseveration   d) alogia

MC/Mod
Pg:412
kind:a
Ans:(b)

12.14: Alogia refers to which aspect of thought disorder?

    a) illogical speech
    b) lack of speech
    c) inability to understand speech
    d) lack of grammatical structure in speech

MC/Mod
Pg:412
kind:f
Ans:(b)

12.15: "Loose associations" refer to which aspect of schizophrenic symptoms?

    a) disruptions in neurotransmitter functioning
    b) social withdrawal and lack of close relationships
    c) illogical jumps in the topic of speech
    d) lack of relation between cognitive and emotional symptoms

MC/Mod
Pg:412
kind:c
Ans:(c)

12.16: Catatonia refers to a disturbance in:

    a) motor functions
    b) speech and thought
    c) emotional expression
    d) capacity for intimacy

MC/Easy
Pg:412
kind:f
Ans:(a)

12.17: Mariella is a schizophrenic patient who is showing
       catatonia. Which of the following behaviors might
       be due to her catatonic condition?

    a) she appears frozen, like a mannequin
    b) she believes she sees her dead father in the
       room
    c) she writes to the CIA about Napoleon's attempts
       to capture her
    d) she answers "Bohemia" to every question asked

MC/Mod
Pg:412
kind:a
Ans:(a)

12.18: Which is true about the state of consciousness
       during a catatonic episode?

    a) the patient appears unaware of surroundings but
       usually is aware
    b) the patient is also delirious
    c) the patient dissociates and will later remember
       nothing
    d) the patient understands very little of what is
       said

MC/Mod
Pg:412
kind:c
Ans:(a)

12.19: Monty, a schizophrenic patient, shows only the
       slightest smile when happy or the slightest frown
       when upset. His emotional expressiveness is
       limited. This is known as:

    a) anhedonia
    b) inappropriate affect
    c) blunted affect
    d) depression

MC/Mod
Pg:412
kind:a
Ans:(c)

12.20: Daniel feels no joy or excitement, even when doing
       things he formerly enjoyed. This symptom is called:

    a) inappropriate affect
    b) blunted affect
    c) anhedonia
    d) affective disorder

MC/Mod
Pg:413
kind:a
Ans:(c)

12.21: Melissa begins giggling when discussing a recent
car accident in which her brother was killed, and
cries when telling a joke she heard on a children's
TV show. This behavior is described as:

    a) anhedonia
    b) inappropriate affect
    c) catatonia
    d) delusional thinking

MC/Mod
Pg:413
kind:a
Ans:(b)

12.22: Avolition refers to:

    a) lack of speech
    b) inappropriate affect
    c) loose associations
    d) indecisiveness and loss of will power

MC/Mod
Pg:413
kind:c
Ans:(d)

12.23: Kraeplin suggested that several types of psychosis
should be distinguished from manic-depressive
disorders and should be classified together under
one category, called:

    a) schizophrenia   b) affective disorder
    c) thought disorder   d) dementia praecox

MC/Mod
Pg:413
kind:f
Ans:(d)

12.24: Bleuler coined the name "schizophrenia" to replace
Kraeplin's term "dementia praecox." The reason
Bleuler wanted a different name was that he
disagreed with the notion, implied by the name
"dementia praecox," that the disorder always:

    a) resulted in memory loss
    b) had an early onset and ended in profound
       deterioration
    c) had a viral cause
    d) involved split personality

MC/Mod
Pg:414
kind:c
Ans:(b)

12.25: Schneider classified certain symptoms of
schizophrenia as "first rank" symptoms. By this he
meant:

    a) early signs of schizophrenia that are
       non-psychotic
    b) symptoms suggesting split personality
    c) specific types of hallucinations and delusions
    d) those indicating dementia

MC/Diff
Pg:414
kind:c
Ans:(c)

12.26: One example of Schneider's first rank symptoms is "thought broadcasting." This is a patient's belief that:

    a) others know what she is thinking
    b) others are forcing her to think a certain way
    c) she knows what others are thinking
    d) she can control what others say about her

MC/Diff
Pg:414
kind:c
Ans:(a)

12.27: European psychiatrists have traditionally used a specific category for patients who experience transient symptoms of schizophrenia and complete recovery. This European diagnosis is:

    a) catatonia
    b) anhedonia
    c) brief reactive psychosis
    d) split personality

MC/Mod
Pg:414
kind:c
Ans:(c)

12.28: The overall impact of changes in the definition of schizophrenia introduced in DSM-III was to:

    a) emphasize the negative symptoms of schizophrenia
    b) emphasize the biological substrates of schizophrenia
    c) broaden the definition of schizophrenia
    d) narrow the definition of schizophrenia

MC/Diff
Pg:415
kind:c
Ans:(d)

12.29: Compared to DSM-III, the DSM-IV definition of schizophrenia places more emphasis on:

    a) negative symptoms
    b) Schneider's first rank symptoms
    c) response to medication
    d) intelligence level

MC/Mod
Pg:415
kind:c
Ans:(a)

12.30: Hebephrenia is now known as which type of schizophrenia?

    a) catatonic   b) paranoid
    c) undifferentiated   d) disorganized

MC/Easy
Pg:416
kind:f
Ans:(d)

12.31: A patient with undifferentiated schizophrenia:

 a) cannot distinguish himself from other people
 b) no longer shows active symptoms of
    schizophrenia
 c) shows unique combinations of psychotic symptoms
    that don't fit any one category
 d) shows the early signs of developing
    schizophrenia

12.32: Schizophrenia of the residual type is found in
people who:

 a) are currently psychotic
 b) were formerly psychotic but continue to have
    problems
 c) are showing the first signs of schizophrenia
 d) inherit the genes for schizophrenia but show no
    symptoms

12.33: Schizoaffective disorder involves:

 a) overlapping periods of psychosis and periods of
    mood disorder
 b) emotionally-based delusions
 c) "cut off" emotions and lack of expressiveness
 d) split personality

12.34: Which of the following must be true for a person to
be diagnosed with delusional disorder rather than
schizophrenia?

 a) there is no history of schizophrenia in the
    family
 b) there are negative, but not positive symptoms
    of schizophrenia
 c) the content of the delusions is not bizarre,
    and there are no other symptoms of schizophrenia
 d) there is evidence of mood disorder

12.35: According to DSM-IV, brief psychotic disorder
refers to psychotic symptoms lasting how long?

 a) less than 24 hours
 b) 1 day to 1 month
 c) 1 month to 6 months
 d) 6 months to 12 months

12.36: Kraeplin's original concept of demential praecox held that all patients with this disorder showed a gradually deteriorating course over the person's lifetime. As conceptualized today, dementia praecox, now called schizophrenia, is thought to take this type of course in about what proportion of patients?

MC/Diff
Pg:417
kind:f
Ans:(b)

a) 5%
c) 50%
b) 30%
d) 75%

12.37: The best predictor of how well an individual will function after a psychotic episode is:

MC/Mod
Pg:418
kind:c
Ans:(c)

a) age
b) gender
c) level of functioning before the episode
d) intelligence

12.38: Most people who develop schizophrenia first show the disorder at what age?

MC/Easy
Pg:418
kind:f
Ans:(b)

a) younger than 15
c) 40-55
b) 15-39
d) over 55

12.39: Studies in the U.S. and Europe show that the lifetime morbid risk of schizophrenia, which is the percentage of the population that will be affected by schizophrenia as some point in their lives, is about:

MC/Mod
Pg:419
kind:f
Ans:(a)

a) 1%
c) 10%
b) 5%
d) 15%

12.40: Cross-cultural studies of the rate of schizophrenia in Western, non-Western, rural, and urban cultures show:

MC/Mod
Pg:419
kind:f
Ans:(d)

a) higher rates in urban areas
b) higher rates in rural areas
c) higher rates in Western cultures
d) similar rates in all areas

12.41: Cross-cultural studies of the rate of schizophrenia in various types of communities found that clinical and social outcomes at 2- and 5-year followup were significantly better in developing countries such as Nigeria and India. This has been interpreted to be a result of which aspect of life in these cultures?

MC/Mod
Pg:419
kind:c
Ans:(a)

a) greater tolerance and acceptance of people with schizophrenia
b) milder forms of schizophrenia
c) racial differences in responses to medication
d) less stressful lifestyles

12.42: Studies of concordance rates for schizophrenia in monozygotic (MZ) and dizygotic (DZ) twins show:

MC/Diff
Pg:420
kind:f
Ans:(b)

a) almost 100% concordance in MZ twins, 0% in DZ
b) consistent evidence of higher concordance in MZ than DZ
c) consistent evidence of higher concordance in DZ than MZ
d) very low rates of concordance in either type of twin

12.43: In order to understand the role of genetics in the development of schizophrenia, researchers have conducted studies of the biological children of schizophrenic mothers, children who are then adopted by non-schizophrenic mothers. Which is true about the rates of schizophrenia among these biological children of schizophrenic mothers?

MC/Diff
Pg:421
kind:c
Ans:(a)

a) same rates if raised by biological mother or adoptive mother
b) higher rates if raised by biological mother
c) lower rates if raised by adoptive mother
d) rates similar to children of non-schizophrenic biological mothers

12.44: Paul Meehl suggested that individuals who are predisposed to schizophrenia inherit a subtle neurological defect of unknown form. He called this condition:

MC/Mod
Pg:424
kind:f
Ans:(b)

a) schizotypy
b) schizotaxia
c) schizophreniform disorder
d) undifferentiated schizophrenia

12.45: According to Meehl's theory of schizotaxia:

    a) all people who show schizotaxia eventually show schizophrenia
    b) schizotaxia is more severe than schizophrenia
    c) schizotaxia is learned; schizophrenia is inherited
    d) mild neurological deficits are associated with a predisposition to schizophrenia

12.46: Structural examination using computerized tomography (CT) scans shows evidence that on average, the brains of schizophrenics have:

    a) enlarged lateral ventricles
    b) enlarged mesocortical pathways
    c) a smaller prefrontal cortex
    d) a smaller cerebellum

12.47: Research evidence to this point indicates that the enlarged lateral ventricles found in schizophrenic patients:

    a) are due to side effects of medication
    b) become more and more enlarged over time
    c) appear early in the development of the disorder
    d) are a transient feature during psychotic episodes

12.48: Research has shown a link between schizophrenia and the lateral ventricles of the brain. Specifically:

    a) all schizophrenics have enlarged lateral ventricles
    b) enlarged lateral ventricles are only found in schizophrenia
    c) on average, schizophrenics have enlarged lateral ventricles
    d) enlarged lateral ventricles predict early onset of schizophrenia

12.49: Magnetic Resonance Imaging (MRI) has found the brains of schizophrenic patients to have smaller sized structures in the:

    a) limbic system   b) prefrontal cortex
    c) corpus callosum   d) cerebellum

12.50: Measures of blood flow in various areas of the   MC/Mod
       cerebral cortex show that while working on abstract   Pg:426
       problem-solving tasks, schizophrenic patients do   kind:f
       not show expected increases in blood flow to: Ans:(c)

           a) the lateral ventricles
           b) the cerebellum
           c) the frontal lobes
           d) the occipital lobes

12.51: The neurological impairments found in schizophrenic   MC/Diff
       patients have also been studied in the unaffected   Pg:426
       twins of schizophrenic patients. Compared to the   kind:c
       neurological impairments of schizophrenic patients,   Ans:(c)
       the neurological impairments in their "well" twins
       are:

           a) the same as in the general population
           b) just as extensive as those of the schizophrenic
              patients
           c) less extensive than the patients', but higher
              than average
           d) more extensive than the patients' impairments

12.52: Studies using Magnetic Resonance Imaging (MRI) have   MC/Diff
       found diminished size of structures in the limbic   Pg:426
       systems of schizophrenics' brains. This may be   kind:f
       important for understanding schizophrenia because   Ans:(c)
       the limbic system is responsible for:

           a) eye tracking and visual perception
           b) abstract reasoning and problem solving
           c) integration of cognition and emotion
           d) consciousness and sense of identity

12.53: The Danish High Risk project found that compared to   MC/Mod
       children in the general population, children of   Pg:427
       schizophrenic parents showed: kind:f
                                                            Ans:(a)

           a) higher rates of schizophrenia
           b) the same rates of schizophrenia as in the
              general population
           c) similar rates of schizophrenia, but higher
              rates of mood disorder
           d) similar rates of schizophrenia, but lower rates
              of mood disorder

12.54: The Danish High Risk project found that compared to
other high risk children who did not develop
schizophrenia, those high risk children who did
develop schizophrenia tended also to have
experienced:

    MC/Mod
    Pg:427
    kind:f
    Ans:(a)

a) prenatal and birth complications
b) exposure to lead in the environment
c) poor nutrition as children
d) early experimentation with alcohol

12.55: Neuroleptics are also known as:

    MC/Easy
    Pg:429
    kind:f
    Ans:(b)

a) neurotransmitters
b) antipsychotic drugs
c) schizophrenic patients
d) brain lesions

12.56: Hypotheses about the etiology of schizophrenia grew
out of attempts to understand how antipsychotic
medications work. Neuroscientists discovered that
animals who received doses of antipsychotic drugs
showed:

    MC/Diff
    Pg:429
    kind:c
    Ans:(b)

a) decreased production of dopamine
b) increased production of dopamine
c) decreased production of serotonin
d) increased production of serotonin

12.57: Patients who receive neuroleptic medication for an
extended period of time often develop side effects
that are similar to those seen in Parkinson's
disease. These motor side effects are thought to
be related to:

    MC/Mod
    Pg:429
    kind:c
    Ans:(c)

a) serotonin deficiency
b) serotonin excess
c) dopamine deficiency
d) dopamine excess

12.58: Amphetamines stimulate firing of dopamine neurons. This provides evidence for the involvement of dopamine in the etiology of schizophrenia, because people who use amphetamines over an extended period of time develop:

MC/Mod
Pg:429
kind:f
Ans:(d)

a) schizotaxia
b) hallucinations
c) avolition and withdrawal
d) paranoia

12.59: Many patients who did not respond to traditional antipsychotics respond to new antipsychotic drugs such as clozapine, which have their biggest effect on:

MC/Easy
Pg:430
kind:f
Ans:(d)

a) dopamine systems
b) acetylcholine levels
c) neuropeptides
d) serotonin systems

12.60: Evidence that the development of schizophrenic disorder is not entirely explained by genetics includes the fact that:

MC/Mod
Pg:430
kind:c
Ans:(c)

a) concordance rates for MZ twins are less than for DZ twins
b) concordance rates for DZ twins are less than for MZ twins
c) MZ twins are not 100% concordant
d) DZ twins are not 100% concordant

12.61: Which of the following describes the relationship between the rate of schizophrenia and social class in the U.S.?

MC/Easy
Pg:430
kind:c
Ans:(c)

a) the highest rates are found in the upper classes
b) the highest rates are found in the middle classes
c) the highest rates are found in the lower classes
d) the rates of schizophrenia are similar across classes

12.62: The social causation hypothesis holds that the high
       rate of schizophrenia in the lower classes in the
       U.S. is due to:

       a) labeling and rejection by society
       b) stressful events and poor health care
       c) high negative emotions in lower class families
       d) inappropriate mothering

MC/Mod
Pg:430
kind:c
Ans:(b)

12.63: According to the social selection hypothesis, the
       rate of schizophrenia is higher in the lower
       classes in the U.S. because:

       a) only poor schizophrenics are labeled as
          mentally ill by society
       b) schizophrenics are less able to finish school
          or hold a good job
       c) the stresses of living in poverty trigger
          schizophrenic symptoms
       d) poor health care and nutrition trigger
          schizophrenic symptoms

MC/Mod
Pg:431
kind:c
Ans:(b)

12.64: Which of the following is evidence that supports
       the social causation hypothesis about the increased
       rates of schizophrenia among the lower classes in
       the U.S.?

       a) periods of high unemployment are followed by
          periods of high psychiatric admission rates
       b) schizophrenics' social status is often lower
          than their fathers'
       c) periods of high unemployment are followed by
          periods of low psychiatric admission rates
       d) schizophrenic persons' social status is often
          higher than their fathers'

MC/Diff
Pg:431
kind:c
Ans:(a)

12.65: Compared to families of nonschizophrenics, the
       families of schizophrenics:

       a) are emotionally cold and uninvolved
       b) are less intelligent
       c) use more severe discipline
       d) have more problems with communication

MC/Mod
Pg:431
kind:f
Ans:(d)

12.66: Interpersonal conflict with family members is thought to influence the:

a) development of schizophrenia
b) the probability of relapse by a schizophrenic patient
c) the content of delusions shown by a schizophrenic patient
d) the display of positive or negative symptoms by schizophrenic patients

MC/Mod
Pg:434
kind:c
Ans:(b)

12.67: "Expressed emotion" has been found to be related to the course of schizophrenia. Expressed emotion refers to:

a) family members being negative and intrusive
b) family members showing acceptance and caring
c) the appropriateness of a schizophrenic person's affect
d) the schizophrenic person's stated desire to engage in social relations

MC/Mod
Pg:434
kind:c
Ans:(a)

12.68: In psychopathology research, groups of schizophrenic patients are sometimes compared to groups of "patient controls." In this case, patient controls are people:

a) without a mental condition
b) predisposed to schizophrenia but not yet showing it
c) who were psychotic in the past but are now in remission
d) with a mental condition other than schizophrenia

MC/Mod
Pg:434
kind:c
Ans:(d)

12.69: Family members often find it hardest to accept and tolerate which aspect of schizophrenic symptoms?

a) hallucinations
b) delusions
c) withdrawal and avolition
d) disorganized speech

MC/Mod
Pg:436
kind:c
Ans:(c)

12.70: One index of vulnerability to schizophrenia may be provided by the Continuous Performance Task. This task is a measure of:

    a) logic skills   b) verbal fluency
    c) attentional skills   d) creativity

MC/Mod
Pg:437
kind:c
Ans:(c)

12.71: Research on the relationship between dysfunctional smooth-pursuit eye movement and schizophrenia has suggested that this dysfunction may be:

    a) a marker for one form of schizophrenia
    b) present in all forms of schizophrenia
    c) not present in the families of schizophrenics
    d) absent in other mental disorders

MC/Mod
Pg:438
kind:c
Ans:(a)

12.72: Many antipsychotic drugs are classified as "neuroleptics" because they:

    a) are also used to treat epilepsy
    b) can produce dementia as side effects
    c) sometimes produce numbness
    d) produce motor side effects like those found in Parkinson's disease

MC/Mod
Pg:439
kind:f
Ans:(d)

12.73: The effectiveness of traditional forms of neuroleptic drugs in reducing psychotic symptoms is directly proportional to their ability to:

    a) increase dopamine production
    b) block dopamine receptors
    c) increase serotonin production
    d) block serotonin receptors

MC/Diff
Pg:439
kind:f
Ans:(b)

12.74: Neuroleptic medications usually produce improvement in psychotic symptoms after about how much time?

    a) within a few hours
    b) after about 2 to 3 days
    c) after several weeks
    d) after about 3 months

MC/Mod
Pg:440
kind:f
Ans:(c)

12.75: Which of the following symptoms is likely to show the most improvement with the use of neuroleptic medication?

    a) alogia   b) hallucinations
    c) blunted affect   d) avolition

MC/Mod
Pg:440
kind:f
Ans:(b)

12.76: About what percentage of schizophrenic patients do NOT respond to traditional neuroleptic medications?

    a) 1%   b) 5%
    c) 25%   d) 50%

MC/Mod
Pg:440
kind:f
Ans:(c)

12.77: Extrapyramidal symptoms are a common side effect of traditional medication used to treat schizophrenia. These symptoms are disturbances in:

    a) attention   b) motor functions
    c) affect regulation d) weight regulation

MC/Mod
Pg:440
kind:f
Ans:(b)

12.78: Scott has been taking neuroleptic medications for years to treat periodic psychosis. Which of the following characterizes the side effects he is most likely to be experiencing?

    a) feels anxious and scared
    b) can't pay attention to TV or reading
    c) involuntarily moves his mouth and hands
    d) has a poor appetite and loses weight

MC/Mod
Pg:440
kind:a
Ans:(c)

12.79: One common problem with prolonged used of traditional neuroleptic medications for treating psychosis is:

    a) schizotaxia   b) tardive dyskinesia
    c) anhedonia   d) alogia

MC/Mod
Pg:440
kind:f
Ans:(b)

12.80: A new class of antipsychotic medications is called "atypical" because these medications:

    a) are used for unusual types of schizophrenia
    b) are usually used for nonschizophrenic disorders
    c) do not produce motor side effects
    d) are effective for a small number of patients

MC/Mod
Pg:441
kind:c
Ans:(c)

12.81: An effective atypical antipsychotic, clozapine, was   MC/Mod
       not approved for use in the U.S. until 1990 because   Pg:441
       it: kind:f
                                                                 Ans:(d)

       a) can be addictive
       b) produces tardive dyskinesia as a side effect
       c) sometimes causes incapacitating anxiety
       d) can produce a lethal blood condition

12.82: Family-based treatment programs that educate family   MC/Mod
       members about schizophrenia and try to reduce   Pg:442
       hostility have been shown to: kind:c
                                                                 Ans:(b)

       a) eliminate relapse
       b) delay relapse
       c) have no effect on relapse
       d) actually speed up relapse

12.83: The social skills deficits of schizophrenic   MC/Mod
       patients are usually: Pg:443
                                                                 kind:c
       a) present only during psychotic episodes   Ans:(c)
       b) correlated with positive symptoms
       c) stable characteristics of these patients
       d) untreatable

12.84: Institutionalized schizophrenics are sometimes   MC/Mod
       helped with the use of token economies. These   Pg:443
       programs are based on: kind:c
                                                                 Ans:(d)
       a) payment for unskilled labor
       b) education about how to manage money
       c) the family paying for treatment, not the state
       d) rewards for appropriate behavior

True-False Questions

12.85: All schizophrenic patients show the same set of   TF/Mod
       core symptoms.   Pg:40(
                                                                 kind:c
                                                                 Ans:False

12.86: All of the symptoms of schizophrenia can also be   TF/Mod
       associated with other psychiatric and medical   Pg:406
       conditions.   kind:c
                                                                 Ans:True

244

12.87: Compared to the prodromal phase of schizophrenia, the residual phase may be characterized by more negative symptoms.

TF/Mod
Pg:408
kind:f
Ans:True

12.88: Auditory hallucinations are the most common form of hallucination experienced by schizophrenic patients.

TF/Easy
Pg:410
kind:f
Ans:True

12.89: The interpersonal relationships of schizophrenics are often characterized by withdrawal and isolation.

TF/Easy
Pg:413
kind:f
Ans:True

12.90: Anhedonia refers to a restricted amount of emotional expressiveness.

TF/Mod
Pg:413
kind:f
Ans:False

12.91: The term "schizophrenia" refers to split personality.

TF/Easy
Pg:414
kind:f
Ans:False

12.92: A person must show evidence of decline in social or occupational functioning in order to be diagnosed with schizophrenia.

TF/Mod
Pg:415
kind:f
Ans:True

12.93: It is unusual for a person to show one subtype of schizophrenia early in life and later show a different subtype of schizophrenia.

TF/Mod
Pg:416
kind:f
Ans:False

12.94: Schizophrenia is much more common in men than in women.

TF/Easy
Pg:418
kind:f
Ans:False

12.95: The gene for schizophrenia has been conclusively located on Chromosome 5.

TF/Mod
Pg:424
kind:f
Ans:False

12.96: Meehl's idea of an inherited neurological defect, called schizotaxia, was based on biological evidence of differences in brain structure and brain functioning in families of schizophrenic patients.

TF/Mod
Pg:425
kind:c
Ans:False

12.97: The neurological impairments found in schizophrenic patients are not found in other mental disorders.

TF/Mod
Pg:428
kind:c
Ans:False

12.98: Traditional types of neuroleptic medications seem to be more beneficial in treating the positive symptoms of schizophrenia than they are in treating the negative symptoms.

TF/Easy
Pg:430
kind:f
Ans:True

12.99: Patterns of expressed emotion among family members of schizophrenics are thought to influence how quickly a schizophrenic patient must return to the hospital.

TF/Mod
Pg:434
kind:c
Ans:True

12.100: Cross-cultural studies of expressed emotion (negativity and intrusiveness in family members of schizophrenics) have found evidence that these attitudes may be more common in non-Western, developing countries.

TF/Mod
Pg:436
kind:c
Ans:False

12.101: One useful index of vulnerability to schizophrenia may be dysfunction in smooth-pursuit eye movement. This dysfunction is most easily measured while a person is dreaming (in REM sleep).

TF/Mod
Pg:438
kind:f
Ans:False

12.102: One of the main effects of the discovery of neuroleptic (antipsychotic) drugs was that many institutionalized patients could be discharged from hospitals.

TF/Mod
Pg:439
kind:c
Ans:True

12.103: Tardive dyskinesia, a side effect of many neuroleptic medications, is eliminated as soon as neuroleptics are discontinued.

TF/Mod
Pg:440
kind:f
Ans:False

12.104: In order to prevent relapse, most schizophrenic   TF/Easy
        patients are prescribed medication on a consistent   Pg:441
        basis, not just while actively psychotic.   kind:f
                                                           Ans:True

Essay Questions

12.105: Delusions are sometimes defined as false beliefs based on incorrect inferences about reality. What is the limitation of this definition? What additional characteristics are important in identifying delusions?

Answer: This definition is limited because it is impossible to define an objective reality. Other factors that must be considered are (1) strong conviction, even when presented with contradictory evidence; (2) preoccupation and inability to avoid thinking about the delusion; (3) lack of perspective or understanding about why others might see the delusion as illogical.

      ES   Moderate   Pages: 411-412   kind: c

12.106: Are gender differences found in schizophrenia? Generally, what are the 2 hypotheses about gender differences in schizophrenia?

Answer: The disorder is equally likely in men and women. However, men show an earlier onset by about 4 or 5 years. This difference may occur because the expression of schizophrenia is mediated by biological factors (e.g. hormones) or social role factors (e.g. stress) that are experienced differently by the two genders. Alternatively, the disorder usually shown by men may be a different disorder than that usually shown by women.

      ES   Moderate   Pages: 419-420   kind: c

12.107: Explain the difference between the social causation hypothesis and the social selection hypothesis in the explanation of higher rates of schizophrenia among the lower classes in the U.S.

Answer: The social causation hypothesis holds that members of the lower classes experience more stressors, which trigger the manifestation of schizophrenia. The social selection hypothesis holds that schizophrenic individuals are less able to complete education and keep a good job, and so their status drifts down to the lower class.

      ES   Moderate   Pages: 430-431   kind: c

12.108: Wynne and Singer observed families of schizophrenic patients interacting in a laboratory and found that parents of schizophrenics show more communication deviance than parents of non-schizophrenics. They concluded that because of interparental conflict and confusing communication patterns, a child is unable to develop a strong identity or the ability to communicate normally, and develops signs of schizophrenia. Describe two alternative explanations for these findings.

Answer: A child who behaves abnormally may elicit changes in parent behavior; evidence for this idea is found in studies showing that normal parents begin to behave differently when interacting with (another family's) schizophrenic child. Alternatively, both the parents and the child could be showing signs of some underlying neurological deficit, which is expressed as schizophrenia by the child but not by the parents; this is Meehl's concept of schizotaxia.

ES   Difficult   Page: 432   kind: c

12.109: What criteria should be met by a potential marker for vulnerability to schizophrenia?

Answer: It should distinguish persons who have schizophrenia from those who do not. It should be a stable characteristic of the individual. It should identify biological relatives at a higher rate than the general population. The trait should be transmitted genetically. It should predict future development of schizophrenia even among the non-psychotic.

ES   Difficult   Page: 437   kind: c

Chapter 13
Dementia, Delirium, and Amnestic Disorders

Multiple Choice Questions

13.1: If allowed to progress, delirium can result in:

    a) Alzheimer's disease   b) dementia
    c) stupor and coma   d) amnestic disorder

MC/Mod
Pg:448
kind:f
Ans:(c)

13.2: Which of the following is characteristic of
    delirium?

    a) usually worse in the daytime
    b) often associated with agitation and
       hyperactivity
    c) acute awareness of one's surroundings
    d) appears gradually over several months

MC/Mod
Pg:448
kind:f
Ans:(b)

13.3: Which of the following is characteristic of
    amnestic disorder?

    a) reduced awareness of one's surroundings
    b) language abilities are unaffected
    c) usually worse at night
    d) reasoning and decision-making abilities are
       impaired

MC/Mod
Pg:448
kind:f
Ans:(b)

13.4: Patients with cognitive disorders are often
    diagnosed and treated by a neurologist. A
    neurologist is:

    a) a psychologist specializing in
       neuropsychological testing
    b) a psychologist specializing in neuroses
    c) a physician specializing in the brain and
       nervous system
    d) a psychiatrist specializing in nervous
       disorders

MC/Easy
Pg:449
kind:f
Ans:(c)

13.5: Dementia and delirium differ in several respects. One difference is that in dementia:

    a) there is a rapid onset
    b) the patient's speech is usually coherent
    c) the patient is unaware of the environment
    d) the problem can be resolved

MC/Mod
Pg:450
kind:c
Ans:(b)

13.6: Jake begins to show delirium while in the hospital. Which of the following is likely to be true of his condition?

    a) his speech is confused
    b) the symptoms of delirium appeared gradually
    c) it is probably a permanent condition
    d) he appears sedated and doesn't show much emotion

MC/Mod
Pg:450
kind:a
Ans:(a)

13.7: The problems associated with dementia are most apparent:

    a) at night
    b) in familiar surroundings
    c) in the patient's speech
    d) in challenging situations

MC/Mod
Pg:450
kind:c
Ans:(d)

13.8: Dementia is an acquired disorder. This means that:

    a) the disorder is transmitted only by virus
    b) the patient's intellectual abilities were previously unimpaired
    c) the patient's previous intellectual abilities were impaired
    d) the disorder has a rapid onset

MC/Mod
Pg:452
kind:f
Ans:(b)

13.9: The most obvious problem during the beginning stages of dementia is:

    a) retrograde amnesia   b) delirium
    c) anterograde amnesia   d) chorea

MC/Diff
Pg:452
kind:f
Ans:(c)

13.10: Mrs. Castillo is in the early stages of dementia.
Which of the following is most characteristic of
the type of problem she is likely to be showing?

    a) her speech doesn't make sense
    b) she shows writhing movements and grimaces
    c) she can't remember the new neighbor she met
       yesterday
    d) she can't remember the name of the town she
       grew up in

MC/Diff
Pg:452
kind:a
Ans:(c)

13.11: Molly suffers a head injury and thereafter cannot
remember anything that happened before the
accident. Her condition is called:

    a) retrograde amnesia   b) anterograde amnesia
    c) agnosia   d) apraxia

MC/Diff
Pg:452
kind:a
Ans:(a)

13.12: In normal development, fluid (problem-solving) and
crystallized (factual) intelligence both develop
continuously over childhood and adolescence. What
changes occur after young adulthood?

    a) fluid intelligence begins to decline
    b) crystallized intelligence begins to decline
    c) both types show gradual declines
    d) crystallized intelligence improves with age

MC/Mod
Pg:453
kind:c
Ans:(a)

13.13: Aphasia refers to various types of loss or
impairment in:

    a) muscle strength and coordination
    b) language abilities
    c) nerve tissue and functioning
    d) neurotransmitter production

MC/Mod
Pg:454
kind:f
Ans:(b)

13.14: The problem in apraxia is that the person:

    a) cannot translate ideas into physical action
    b) cannot understand speech
    c) has muscles that are too weak to move
    d) forgets the names of objects

MC/Diff
Pg:454
kind:c
Ans:(a)

13.15: The problem in visual agnosia is that the person:

    a) has a sensory deficit and cannot see
    b) knows what an object is for, but not its name
    c) cannot move the mouth muscles to name an object
    d) does not recognize an object as something
       meaningful

MC/Diff
Pg:455
kind:c
Ans:(d)

13.16: A psychologist holds out a comb and asks Mr. Bonte "What is this called in my hand?" Mr. Bonte replies, "I have no idea what that's called." The psychologist then asks Mr. Bonte to show what he would do with the object. Mr. Bonte says, "How should I know? I don't know what it is!" Mr. Bonte's response led the psychologist to describe his condition as:

    a) aphasia   b) agnosia
    c) apraxia   d) Alzheimer's disease

MC/Diff
Pg:455
kind:a
Ans:(b)

13.17: "Halstead Reitan" is the name of a:

    a) form of dementia
    b) treatment center for Alzheimer's disease
       patients
    c) microscopic technique for assessing brain
       tissue damage
    d) neuropsychological test battery

MC/Easy
Pg:456
kind:f
Ans:(d)

13.18: The Mini-Mental State Exam assesses:

    a) clinicians' qualifications as neurologists
    b) a patient's emotions and level of depression
    c) microscopic lesions in the brain
    d) cognitive functioning

MC/Easy
Pg:456
kind:f
Ans:(d)

13.19: Ms. Duglet shows dyskinesia. Which of the following is most likely to happen due to her condition?

    a) she might accidentally knock over a lamp
    b) she might not be able to think of the word
       "lamp"
    c) she might not remember buying a lamp
    d) she might get excessively angry because she
       dislikes a new lamp

MC/Mod
Pg:457
kind:a
Ans:(a)

13.20: Dyskinesia is associated with some types of dementia. Dyskinesia is a symptom characterized by:

a) involuntary movements
b) inability to name objects
c) loss of memory for past events
d) exaggerated emotionality

MC/Mod
Pg:457
kind:f
Ans:(a)

13.21: A type of amnestic disorder associated with chronic alcoholism is:

a) Alzheimer's disease
b) Huntington's disease
c) Korsakoff's syndrome
d) Pick's disease

MC/Easy
Pg:459
kind:f
Ans:(c)

13.22: Korsakoff's syndrome is considered to be an amnestic disorder because:

a) delirium is a common symptom
b) abilities for abstract thinking are impaired
c) there is associated dyskinesia
d) memory is impaired but other cognitive functions are not

MC/Mod
Pg:459
kind:c
Ans:(d)

13.23: One theory regarding the etiology of Korsakoff's syndrome is:

a) vitamin deficiency due to poor diet
b) disruption of neurotransmitter functioning
c) head injury while intoxicated
d) chronic electrolyte imbalance due to vomiting

MC/Mod
Pg:459
kind:c
Ans:(a)

13.24: Korsakoff's syndrome is thought to be caused by damage to which part of the brain?

a) Broca's area   b) medial thalamus
c) Wernicke's area   d) frontal lobe

MC/Diff
Pg:459
kind:f
Ans:(b)

13.25: Paul Broca, a French surgeon (1824-1880), demonstrated that lesions in the left frontal lobe are associated with a specific type of:

a) apraxia   b) dementia
c) amnesia   d) aphasia

MC/Mod
Pg:460
kind:c
Ans:(d)

13.26: Carl Wernicke, a German neurologist (1848-1905), identified a specific form of aphasia associated with damage to the:

MC/Diff
Pg:460
kind:f
Ans:(a)

    a) posterior cortex   b) left frontal lobe
    c) hippocampus   d) medial thalamus

13.27: An important step in the identification of dementias was the discovery of bundles of neurofibrillary tangles and senile plaques in the brains of deceased dementia patients. This discovery was made by:

MC/Mod
Pg:460
kind:f
Ans:(a)

    a) Alzheimer   b) Kraeplin
    c) Korsakoff   d) Pinel

13.28: Emil Kraeplin is known for:

MC/Mod
Pg:460
kind:c
Ans:(c)

    a) microscopic analysis of the brain tissue of dementia patients
    b) demonstrating memory loss due to lesions in the medial thalamus
    c) writing a textbook classifying psychiatric disorders
    d) identifying areas of brain damage associated with aphasia

13.29: Emil Kraeplin distinguished between early-onset dementia and senile dementia. By senile dementia, he meant a dementia characterized by:

MC/Mod
Pg:460
kind:c
Ans:(a)

    a) onset after age 65
    b) worse memory loss
    c) delirium
    d) more brain pathology

13.30: In the DSM-IV, dementias are classified as:

MC/Mod
Pg:460
kind:f
Ans:(b)

    a) organic mental disorders
    b) cognitive disorders
    c) deliria
    d) amnestic disorders

13.31: By definition, a primary dementia is characterized by:

MC/Mod
Pg:461
kind:c
Ans:(d)

a) disturbances of muscle control
b) memory loss but no language impairment
c) impairment due to something other than brain disease
d) impairment due to the direct effect of brain disease

13.32: Dementias due to treatable illnesses such as vascular disease, infections, and substance abuse are known as:

MC/Mod
Pg:461
kind:c
Ans:(c)

a) undifferentiated   b) differentiated
c) secondary   d) primary

13.33: Huntington's disease and Parkinson's disease have in common:

MC/Mod
Pg:461
kind:f
Ans:(b)

a) alcohol abuse
b) disturbances in muscular control
c) dementia in all cases
d) apraxia and aphasia

13.34: Alzheimer's disease and Pick's disease are called "undifferentiated" dementias because:

MC/Mod
Pg:461
kind:c
Ans:(c)

a) their symptoms are too variable to classify
b) the underlying biological causes are the same
c) their manifest symptoms are the same
d) they are associated with significant muscular impairment

13.35: Which of the following is necessary for a diagnosis of dementia?

MC/Mod
Pg:461
kind:c
Ans:(b)

a) muscular impairment
b) impairment in social or occupational functioning
c) language impairment
d) delirium

13.36: Alzheimer's disease is distinguished from other types of dementia in DSM-IV based on:

   a) more significant memory impairment
   b) gradual speed on onset
   c) muscular impairment
   d) personality changes

MC/Mod
Pg:461
kind:f
Ans:(b)

13.37: Patients with cognitive disorders are often tested with implicit memory tasks. These tasks are designed so that a subject who does the task:

   a) is specifically told to try to remember something
   b) is asked about things that were learned years earlier
   c) is asked to remember how they solved a problem
   d) might learn something without trying

MC/Mod
Pg:462
kind:c
Ans:(d)

13.38: Psychologists studied the case of R.B., a man who developed cognitive impairments after the blood supply to his brain was interrupted during surgery, in order to learn more about the brain mechanisms responsible for cognitive functions. In the case of R.B., testing and autopsy provided information on the link between:

   a) memory impairment and damage to the hippocampus
   b) memory impairment and damage to the medial thalamus
   c) language impairment and damage to the cerebellum
   d) language impairment and damage to the basal ganglia

MC/Mod
Pg:462
kind:f
Ans:(a)

13.39: Which of the following is a result that has been found in laboratory tests in which normal elderly persons, Alzheimer's patients, and patients with Huntington's disease are asked to engage in implicit memory tasks?

   a) Alzheimer's patients show worse verbal implicit memory
   b) Huntington's patients show worse verbal implicit memory
   c) Alzheimer's and Huntington's patients both show worse motor implicit memory
   d) Alzheimer's and Huntington's patients show no deficits in implicit memory

MC/Mod
Pg:463
kind:f
Ans:(a)

13.40: Which of the following characterizes the
neurofibrils of the neurons in the brains of
Alzheimer's patients?

    a) they have a core of amyloid
    b) they are missing
    c) they are symmetrical
    d) they are disorganized

MC/Diff
Pg:463
kind:f
Ans:(d)

13.41: Alzheimer's disease is associated with
abnormalities of the neurofibrils. Neurofibrils
are important for:

    a) functioning of the basal ganglia
    b) dopamine reuptake in the substantia nigra
    c) cell structure and production of
       neurotransmitters
    d) transportation of oxygen to the brain

MC/Diff
Pg:463
kind:f
Ans:(c)

13.42: Patients with Alzheimer's, Down Syndrome, and
Parkinson's disease have all been shown to have:

    a) an extra chromosome
    b) degeneration of the substantia nigra
    c) neurofibrillary tangles
    d) Pick's bodies

MC/Diff
Pg:463
kind:c
Ans:(c)

13.43: Senile plaques are essentially:

    a) asymmetrical neurofibrils
    b) clumps of debris from dead neurons
    c) ballooning of nerve cells
    d) clogged arteries to the brain

MC/Mod
Pg:463
kind:f
Ans:(b)

13.44: A dementia that is very similar to Alzheimer's
disease, but which also often involves early
personality changes, disinhibition, and aimless
exploration, is:

    a) Huntington's disease
    b) Parkinson's disease
    c) vascular dementia
    d) Pick's disease

MC/Diff
Pg:464
kind:c
Ans:(d)

13.45: Pick's bodies are:

    a) tangles of neurofibrils
    b) bunches of dead neurons
    c) asymmetrical cell bodies
    d) distinctive ballooning of brain cells

MC/Mod
Pg:464
kind:f
Ans:(d)

13.46: Chorea is a symptom of:

    a) Alzheimer's disease
    b) Parkinson's disease
    c) Huntington's disease
    d) vascular dementia

MC/Easy
Pg:464
kind:f
Ans:(c)

13.47: Mr. Edthorpe shows Huntington's chorea. Which of
the following would he have most trouble doing?

    a) knowing that the name of a comb is "comb"
    b) knowing his hair was messy and needed to be
       combed
    c) combing his hair
    d) knowing what a comb was for

MC/Mod
Pg:464
kind:a
Ans:(c)

13.48: The cognitive and motor deficits associated with
Huntington's disease are due to neuronal
degeneration in the:

    a) basal ganglia   b) medial thalamus
    c) hippocampus   d) frontal lobe

MC/Diff
Pg:464
kind:f
Ans:(a)

13.49: Parkinson's disease is MOST characterized by:

    a) chorea   b) tremors
    c) aphasia   d) dementia

MC/Mod
Pg:464
kind:c
Ans:(b)

13.50: One of the leading causes of secondary dementia is:

    a) Parkinson's disease
    b) Huntington's disease
    c) blood vessel disease
    d) Alzheimer's disease

MC/Mod
Pg:464
kind:f
Ans:(c)

13.51: A stroke occurs when:

   a) the heart stops beating
   b) a seizure disrupts neuronal transmissions
   c) blood flow to the brain is interrupted
   d) head injury causes damage to the frontal lobe
      area

MC/Easy
Pg:465
kind:f
Ans:(c)

13.52: Marla is unable to move the right side of her body,
       but the other side of her body is mobile. A likely
       cause of this problem is:

   a) stroke
   b) Parkinson's disease
   c) neurofibrillary tangles
   d) Pick's disease

MC/Mod
Pg:465
kind:a
Ans:(a)

13.53: An infarct is:

   a) dementia due to depression
   b) a clogged artery to the brain
   c) a surgical procedure to clean brain plaque
   d) an area of dead brain tissue caused by a stroke

MC/Mod
Pg:465
kind:f
Ans:(d)

13.54: Vascular dementia is also known as:

   a) Parkinson's disease
   b) Huntington's disease
   c) multi-infarct dementia
   d) Korsakoff's syndrome

MC/Easy
Pg:465
kind:f
Ans:(c)

13.55: Multi-infarct dementia and Alzheimer's disease have
       the same:

   a) cause
   b) cognitive impairments
   c) rate of onset
   d) motor impairments

MC/Diff
Pg:465
kind:c
Ans:(b)

13.56: "Pseudodementia" refers to a condition in which:

   a) the memory loss is not severe
   b) there is no motor impairment
   c) cognitive impairment is produced by major
      depression
   d) the symptoms are faked

MC/Mod
Pg:466
kind:c
Ans:(c)

13.57: In the near future, the number of new cases of dementia in the U.S. is expected to be:

a) higher, because the population is aging
b) higher, because of increased toxins in the environment
c) lower, because of new technology that has been discovered for prevention
d) lower, because of new medications that have been shown to be effective treatments

MC/Easy
Pg:466
kind:f
Ans:(a)

13.58: The average time between onset of Alzheimer's disease and the person's death is:

a) a few months
b) 1 year
c) 8 years
d) 20 years

MC/Mod
Pg:467
kind:f
Ans:(c)

13.59: Men show higher rates of dementia due to:

a) Alzheimer's disease
b) vascular disease
c) Pick's disease
d) Huntington's disease

MC/Mod
Pg:467
kind:f
Ans:(b)

13.60: The rarest form of dementia is:

a) Alzheimer's disease
b) Pick's disease
c) Huntington's disease
d) vascular disease

MC/Mod
Pg:467
kind:f
Ans:(c)

13.61: The most common form of dementia is:

a) Pick's disease
b) vascular disease
c) Huntington's disease
d) Alzheimer's disease

MC/Easy
Pg:467
kind:f
Ans:(d)

13.62: In studies of extended families in which some members are affected by a disease and other members are unaffected by it, which of the following must be established in order to identify genetic linkage?

  a) family members affected by the disease do not have the marker
  b) family members with the disease have the marker; unaffected members do not have the marker
  c) both affected and unaffected members have the marker
  d) the marker is only present in one family and not in other families

13.63: An autosomal trait is one associated with a gene that:

  a) is not on one of the sex chromosomes
  b) is on one of the sex chromosomes
  c) is not linked with a marker
  d) has mutated

13.64: Senile plaques and neurofibrillary tangles, typical in Alzheimer's disease, are also found in all patients with:

  a) Korsakoff's syndrome
  b) Parkinson's disease
  c) Schizophrenia
  d) Down syndrome

13.65: Alzheimer's patients and Down syndrome patients have what in common?

  a) low intelligence
  b) agitation
  c) senile plaques and neurofibrillary tangles
  d) dopamine deficiency

13.66: Genetic linkage analysis refers to:

  a) locating a gene that is responsible for a disorder or trait
  b) documenting patterns of inheritance in families
  c) microscopic analysis of nerve cell damage
  d) educating family members about chances of inheritance

13.67: Creutzfeldt-Jakob disease is thought to be caused by:

    a) overexposure to aluminum
    b) dopamine deficiency
    c) a slow-acting virus
    d) an abnormality on chromosome 21

MC/Mod
Pg:469
kind:f
Ans:(c)

13.68: It has been hypothesized that Alzheimer's disease and immune system dysfunction are related. This hypothesis is based on evidence that patients with both these disorders show:

    a) amyloid in dead brain tissue
    b) high levels of aluminum in their bodies
    c) trisomy 21
    d) dopamine deficiency

MC/Mod
Pg:470
kind:c
Ans:(a)

13.69: Although controversial, some research suggests an association between Alzheimer's disease and exposure to high levels of:

    a) copper   b) radioactivity
    c) carbon monoxide d) aluminum

MC/Easy
Pg:470
kind:f
Ans:(d)

13.70: Which of the following has the best chance for successful treatment and recovery?

    a) Down syndrome   b) delirium
    c) primary dementia d) secondary dementia

MC/Diff
Pg:471
kind:c
Ans:(b)

13.71: Medication to improve the immediate signs and symptoms of Alzheimer-type dementia is designed to increase levels of:

    a) acetylcholine   b) dopamine
    c) serotonin   d) amyloid

MC/Diff
Pg:471
kind:f
Ans:(a)

13.72: About 80% of patients with Alzheimer's dementia:

    a) are cared for by spouses and family members
    b) are institutionalized
    c) live alone
    d) do not need any special assistance

MC/Mod
Pg:472
kind:f
Ans:(a)

13.73: Respite programs are designed to provide:

    a) prescription drugs for impoverished dementia patients
    b) financial assistance for dementia patients
    c) a spa-like living atmosphere for dementia patients
    d) assistance for the caretakers of dementia patients

MC/Easy
Pg:473
kind:f
Ans:(d)

True-False Questions

13.74: Dementia is a gradual worsening of memory and other cognitive functions.

TF/Easy
Pg:448
kind:f
Ans:True

13.75: The memory impairment in amnestic disorders is usually more extensive than that found in delerium or dementia.

TF/Mod
Pg:448
kind:f
Ans:False

13.76: A neurologist is a psychologist who specializes in neuropsychological testing.

TF/Easy
Pg:449
kind:f
Ans:False

13.77: Although dementia is associated with severe impairment of memory and other cognitive functions, the patient's personality and emotions are generally unaffected.

TF/Mod
Pg:450
kind:c
Ans:False

13.78: By definition, dementia affects cognitive functioning but not motor functioning.

TF/Mod
Pg:452
kind:f
Ans:False

13.79: A person with apraxia understands instructions but lacks the coordination and muscle strength to follow them.

TF/Mod
Pg:454
kind:f
Ans:False

13.80: A person with aphasia cannot name an object, but can show what the object is used for.

TF/Diff
Pg:454
kind:f
Ans:True

13.81: If hallucinations or delusions are present, a diagnosis of dementia is not made.

TF/Mod
Pg:457
kind:c
Ans:False

13.82: In amnestic disorders, there is severe impairment of memory but higher level cognitive abilities are unaffected.

TF/Easy
Pg:458
kind:f
Ans:True

13.83: Dementias used to be classified as organic mental disorders.

TF/Mod
Pg:460
kind:f
Ans:True

13.84: Microscopic analysis of brain tissue is necessary to diagnose undifferentiated dementias with certainty.

TF/Mod
Pg:461
kind:f
Ans:True

13.85: Laboratory learning tasks are able to detect average differences in the type of cognitive impairments seen in Alzheimer's disease and Huntington's disease, even though such differences are difficult to detect clinically.

TF/Mod
Pg:462
kind:c
Ans:True

13.86: The brains of people over the age of 75 often have some neurofibrillary tangles and senile plaques.

TF/Easy
Pg:463
kind:f
Ans:True

13.87: All patients with Huntington's disease eventually show dementia.

TF/Mod
Pg:464
kind:f
Ans:True

13.88: Almost all patients with Parkinson's disease show dementia.

TF/Mod
Pg:464
kind:f
Ans:False

13.89: People with an earlier onset of Alzheimer's disease usually survive for a longer period than people with a later onset.

TF/Mod
Pg:467
kind:f
Ans:False

13.90: All cases of Alzheimer's disease are due to an inherited gene located on chromosome 21.

TF/Mod
Pg:469
kind:f
Ans:False

13.91: If a dementia disorder runs in families, then a viral cause can be ruled out.

TF/Mod
Pg:469
kind:c
Ans:False

13.92: Many conditions that cause delirium can be treated, eliminating the delirium.

TF/Mod
Pg:471
kind:f
Ans:True

13.93: It is important to keep Alzheimer's patients physically active because such activity reduces agitation and improves sleep.

TF/Mod
Pg:472
kind:c
Ans:True

Essay Questions

13.94: Describe the emotional changes that may accompany dementia.

Answer: The affect of dementia patients can be flat, with an apathetic appearance. However, emotional expression can also become exaggerated and less predictable. Depression often accompanies dementia.

ES Moderate Page: 457 kind: c

13.95: Explain the difference between undifferentiated dementias and differentiated dementias. How is each type diagnosed?

Answer: Undifferentiated dementias (such as Alzheimer's disease and Pick's disease) have similar symptoms that cannot be easily distinguished clinically. Their diagnosis depends on post-mortem microscopic analysis of the brain, which shows different underlying brain abnormalities. Differentiated dementias (such as Huntington's disease and Parkinson's disease) show clearly different symptoms, especially motor symptoms, which are easily noted clinically. Therefore their diagnosis can be made without post-mortem analysis of brain tissue.

ES Moderate Page: 461 kind: c

13.96: Explain why it is difficult for epidemiologists to get an accurate picture of the number of cases of dementia, and the types of dementia, in the U.S. population.

Answer: Generally the epidemiologists' problem is one of diagnosis. Mild symptoms of dementia are difficult to distinguish from problems associated with normal aging. Mild symptoms are hard to detect reliably. In order to diagnose dementia, multiple assessments are required over time, whereas epidemiological assessments are usually made at one time point. Finally, the undifferentiated dementias require post-mortem analysis of brain tissue to make an accurate diagnosis of a specific type of dementia.

ES Moderate Page: 466 kind: c

13.97: Describe what chromosome 21 has to do with our understanding of Alzheimer's disease and Down syndrome.

Answer: Down syndrome is associated with trisomy 21 (having 3 copies of chromosome 21 rather than 2). Down syndrome and Alzheimer's disease patients both have neurofibrillary tangles and senile plaque in brain tissue. This similarity led researchers to search for a gene for Alzheimer's on chromosome 21, the source of the abnormalities in Down syndrome. Such a gene has been located for the Alzheimer's disease found in some families, but not all families. It appears that the gene responsible for the production of proteins used to make amyloid (the core of senile plaques) is located on chromosome 21.

ES Moderate Page: 468 kind: c

13.98: Describe the ways that a demented person's environment can be constructed to minimize the patient's distress.

Answer: Labeling rooms and other parts of the environment, since the patient cannot remember directions and may get lost; arranging rooms so that spaces that the patient uses are visible from his or her room, since the patient may forget about these other areas or get lost; make sure the environment is secure, so that the patient does not wander off.

ES Moderate Page: 472 kind: a

Chapter 14
Mental Retardation and
Pervasive Developmental Disorders

Multiple Choice Questions

14.1: Which of the following do Mental Retardation and Pervasive Developmental Disorder have in common?

    a) caused by chromosomal defect
    b) inability to live independently
    c) disinterest in relationships
    d) present at birth or onset in childhood

MC/Easy
Pg:478
kind:c
Ans:(d)

14.2: Which condition usually accompanies Pervasive Developmental Disorder?

    a) sensory deficits
    b) savant abilities
    c) mental retardation
    d) motor incoordination

MC/Mod
Pg:478
kind:f
Ans:(c)

14.3: Brenda is 29 and has an IQ of 67. She finished 4th grade. She lives with her boyfriend and pays her bills with money she earns as a farm laborer. She is well able to live without supervision. In terms of the classification of Mental Retardation (MR) according to the DSM-IV, Brenda:

    a) would be considered MR because of low IQ
    b) would be considered MR because of low educational status
    c) would not be considered MR, because she's functioning adaptively
    d) would not be considered MR, because she is over 18

MC/Mod
Pg:480
kind:a
Ans:(c)

14.4: According to the DSM-IV, Mental Retardation is diagnosed if low IQ and concurrent deficits in adaptive functioning:

    a) are unrelated to biological causes
    b) are present before the age of 18
    c) have been present more than 1 year
    d) are considered irreversible

MC/Mod
Pg:480
kind:c
Ans:(b)

14.5: When factors such as injury or degenerative brain disease produce subaverage IQs and related deficits in adaptive functioning in someone older than 18, the person is not given the diagnosis of Mental Retardation. Instead, the diagnosis is likely to be:

MC/Mod
Pg:480
kind:c
Ans:(a)

    a) dementia   b) delirium
    c) Asperger's disorder   d) cortical trauma

14.6: According to the American Association for the Mentally Retarded (AAMR), a person can only be diagnosed as Mentally Retarded if their IQ is below:

MC/Easy
Pg:480
kind:f
Ans:(c)

    a) 25   b) 50
    c) 75   d) 100

14.7: The system used in early intelligence tests to derive IQ is no longer used. According to this system, IQ was calculated by:

MC/Mod
Pg:481
kind:c
Ans:(c)

    a) comparing a score to group norms
    b) translating a score into standard deviations
    c) dividing the mental age by the chronological age
    d) dividing the chronological age by the mental age

14.8: Most intelligence tests are standardized to have:

MC/Easy
Pg:481
kind:f
Ans:(d)

    a) a mean of 85 and a standard deviation of 15
    b) a mean of 115 and a standard deviation of 30
    c) a mean of 100 and a standard deviation of 30
    d) a mean of 100 and a standard deviation of 15

14.9: The cutoff score for Mental Retardation is approximately 2 standard deviations below the mean. If IQ scores were normally distributed, this would mean theoretically that about what percentage of the population would fall below this cutoff?

MC/Mod
Pg:481
kind:f
Ans:(b)

    a) 0.5 %   b) 2-3 %
    c) 7 %   d) 10 %

14.10: Which of the following children is most likely to show a significant change in IQ score if retested 5 years later?

    a) a 4-year-old   b) a 10-year-old
    c) a 13-year-old   d) a 17-year-old

MC/Mod
Pg:481
kind:a
Ans:(a)

14.11: IQ tests are best used for the purpose for which they were designed, which is:

    a) as an indicator of adaptive functioning
    b) to rank people according to intelligence
    c) to detect the extraordinarily gifted
    d) as a measure of potential for school achievement

MC/Mod
Pg:481
kind:c
Ans:(d)

14.12: In addition to an IQ test, which of the following tests might be used to make a diagnosis of Mental Retardation?

    a) Halstead Reitan Neuropsychological Battery
    b) Minnesota Multiphasic Personality Inventory
    c) Scholastic Aptitude Test
    d) Vineland Adaptive Behavior Scales

MC/Easy
Pg:482
kind:c
Ans:(d)

14.13: Which of the following events would be the most LIKELY reason that a person formerly classified as mentally retarded would no longer be classified as mentally retarded 1 year later?

    a) the person turned 18
    b) the person's IQ increased significantly
    c) the person functions more independently at work than at school
    d) the person became financially independent

MC/Mod
Pg:482
kind:c
Ans:(c)

14.14: Whether a person is considered mentally retarded depends in part on the culture's definition of mental retardation. Specifically, cultures vary in terms of:

    a) their understanding of genetic abnormalities
    b) their recognition that mental retardation is not insanity
    c) the importance of academic aptitude for success
    d) the use of standardized IQ tests

MC/Mod
Pg:483
kind:c
Ans:(c)

14.15: Itard's work with the "wild boy of Aveyron," found living in the woods in 1799, was important because it:

MC/Mod
Pg:483
kind:c
Ans:(a)

a) spurred interest in special education for the mentally retarded
b) showed that even severe intellectual deficits can be overcome
c) established an environmental cause of mental retardation
d) established a genetic cause of mental retardation

14.16: In 1866 British physician Langdon Down first described:

MC/Easy
Pg:483
kind:f
Ans:(a)

a) a subgroup of mental retardation
b) the case of the "wild boy of Aveyron"
c) the characteristics of autism
d) the condition of pervasive developmental disorder

14.17: In 1905 Binet and Simon developed the first intelligence test in response to a request by the French government to identify:

MC/Easy
Pg:483
kind:f
Ans:(d)

a) the extraordinarily gifted
b) men fit for the military
c) civil service personnel needing further training
d) children in need of special education

14.18: The first IQ test was developed by:

MC/Easy
Pg:483
kind:f
Ans:(d)

a) Itard
b) Kanner
c) Down
d) Binet and Simon

14.19: According to the DSM-IV, MILD Mental Retardation is a designation for people with deficits in adaptive functioning and with IQs between:

MC/Mod
Pg:484
kind:f
Ans:(b)

a) 35-50
b) 50-70
c) 70-85
d) 85-100

14.20: What percentage of the mentally retarded are classified as MILDLY mentally retarded?

MC/Easy
Pg:484
kind:f
Ans:(d)

a) 3%
b) 15%
c) 50%
d) 85%

14.21: The vast majority of the mentally retarded are classified as mildly mentally retarded. These persons typically achieve which level of academic functioning?

MC/Mod
Pg:484
kind:f
Ans:(c)

a) kindergarten
b) 2nd grade
c) 6th grade
d) 10th grade

14.22: The smallest number of mentally retarded fall in which category of mental retardation?

MC/Mod
Pg:484
kind:f
Ans:(d)

a) mild
b) moderate
c) severe
d) profound

14.23: The most common known biological cause of mental retardation is:

MC/Mod
Pg:485
kind:f
Ans:(a)

a) Down syndrome
b) fragile X syndrome
c) PKU
d) lead poisoning

14.24: Which of the following typifies mental retardation due to known biological origin?

MC/Mod
Pg:485
kind:c
Ans:(b)

a) it is milder than other forms of mental retardation
b) it is more commonly associated with physical handicaps
c) it is more common among the poor and lower classes
d) it accounts for 85% of mental retardation

14.25: Trisomy 21, the presence of an extra chromosome on the 21st pair, is another name for:

MC/Easy
Pg:486
kind:f
Ans:(c)

a) fragile X syndrome
b) Kanner's syndrome
c) Down syndrome
d) Turner syndrome

14.26: The incidence of Down syndrome is related to:

    a) maternal alcohol use during pregnancy
    b) presence of the disorder in the parents
    c) maternal age
    d) environmental toxins

MC/Mod
Pg:486
kind:f
Ans:(c)

14.27: A recent discovery in the study of Down syndrome is that by their 30s, these patients develop brain pathology similar to that found in:

    a) Parkinson's disease
    b) Alzheimer's disease
    c) Huntington's disease
    d) Korsakoff's syndrome

MC/Easy
Pg:486
kind:f
Ans:(b)

14.28: Fragile X syndrome is characterized by:

    a) an abnormality on the X sex chromosome
    b) an extra Y sex chromosome
    c) an extra X sex chromosome
    d) a missing X sex chromosome

MC/Easy
Pg:486
kind:f
Ans:(a)

14.29: XYY syndrome was once thought to be associated with:

    a) homosexuality   b) criminality
    c) schizophrenia   d) autism

MC/Mod
Pg:486
kind:f
Ans:(b)

14.30: Which of the following only occurs in females?

    a) Turner syndrome
    b) fragile X syndrome
    c) Klinefelter syndrome
    d) XYY syndrome

MC/Mod
Pg:487
kind:f
Ans:(a)

14.31: Children with PKU develop mental retardation because of:

    a) malnutrition
    b) chromosomal abnormalities
    c) head injury
    d) unmetabolized phenylalanine

MC/Mod
Pg:487
kind:c
Ans:(d)

14.32: The mental retardation associated with PKU can   MC/Mod
       often be diminished dramatically if the child: Pg:487
                                                                kind:f
       a) undergoes long-term behavior modification   Ans:(b)
       b) eats foods low in phenylalanine
       c) can be taught sign language
       d) gets a blood transfusion

14.33: A genetic disorder that is more common among Jewish   MC/Mod
       people of Eastern European heritage than among   Pg:487
       other ethnic groups is: kind:f
                                                                Ans:(a)
       a) Tay-Sachs disease
       b) Turner syndrome
       c) PKU
       d) Klinefelter syndrome

14.34: A rare recessive gene disorder often associated   MC/Mod
       with mental retardation and gross physical   Pg:487
       abnormalities including gargoylism is: kind:f
                                                                Ans:(c)
       a) Klinefelter's syndrome
       b) Turner syndrome
       c) Hurler syndrome
       d) PKU

14.35: Lesch-Nyman syndrome is a rare gene disorder   MC/Mod
       associated with mental retardation and notable for   Pg:487
       accompanying: kind:f
                                                                Ans:(a)
       a) self-mutilating behavior
       b) disturbed eating habits
       c) gross physical abnormalities
       d) criminality

14.36: A child can be born with severe mental retardation   MC/Mod
       if the mother contracts Rubella (German measles):   Pg:487
                                                                kind:f
       a) in the first trimester   Ans:(a)
       b) in the second trimester
       c) in the third trimester
       d) right before and during delivery

14.37: A disease that can result in mental retardation in   MC/Mod
children and that can be transmitted from the   Pg:488
mother to the child during the delivery is: kind:f
                                                         Ans:(c)

    a) rubella   b) syphilis
    c) genital herpes   d) encephalitis

14.38: Which of the following causes of mental retardation   MC/Mod
is due to infection of the brain?   Pg:488
                                                         kind:c
    a) encephalitis   Ans:(a)
    b) fetal alcohol syndrome
    c) PKU
    d) Klinefelter syndrome

14.39: Fetal alcohol syndrome is associated with retarded   MC/Mod
physical development and: Pg:488
                                                         kind:c
    a) mild mental retardation and learning   Ans:(a)
       disabilities
    b) moderate mental retardation
    c) severe mental retardation
    d) profound mental retardation

14.40: The use of heroin, methadone, and crack by pregnant   MC/Mod
women puts their babies at high risk for: Pg:488
                                                         kind:f
    a) chromosomal abnormalities   Ans:(d)
    b) PKU
    c) brain infection
    d) low birthweight

14.41: Exposure to high levels of lead can lead to mental   MC/Easy
retardation. One common cause of lead exposure in   Pg:489
children is: kind:f
                                                         Ans:(a)
    a) chips of lead-based paint
    b) lead plumbing and pipes
    c) canned foods
    d) insulation

14.42: The problem in Rh incompatibility during pregnancy is that:

    a) unmetabolized amino acids cause brain damage
    b) the mother's antibodies attack the fetus' blood cells
    c) brain infection causes damaging cranial pressure
    d) chromosomal abnormalities cause retardation

MC/Mod
Pg:489
kind:c
Ans:(b)

14.43: Cultural-familial retardation describes mental retardation that is due to:

    a) chromosomal abnormalities common in certain ethnic groups
    b) sexually transmitted diseases
    c) drug abuse during pregnancy
    d) a combination of poverty and inherited intelligence

MC/Mod
Pg:489
kind:c
Ans:(d)

14.44: Which of the following pairs of relatives show the highest correlation in IQ scores?

    a) identical twins reared apart
    b) biological siblings reared together
    c) biological parent and child
    d) adoptive parent and child

MC/Diff
Pg:489
kind:c
Ans:(a)

14.45: In contrast to mental retardation caused by conditions like PKU, cultural-familial retardation is due to:

    a) the effects of a single gene, not multiple genes
    b) factors other than nutrition
    c) the effects of multiple genes, not one gene
    d) chromosomal abnormality

MC/Mod
Pg:489
kind:c
Ans:(c)

14.46: Cultural-familial retardation is found far more frequently among the poor, in part because:

    a) chromosomal abnormalities are more common in the lower classes
    b) poor nutrition causes PKU
    c) impoverished environments can be less intellectually stimulating
    d) sexually transmitted diseases are more common in the lower classes

MC/Mod
Pg:491
kind:c
Ans:(c)

14.47: Which of the following is most likely to be
associated with conditions of poverty such as poor
nutrition and lack of educational materials?

a) mild mental retardation
b) moderate mental retardation
c) severe mental retardation
d) profound mental retardation

MC/Diff
Pg:491
kind:c
Ans:(a)

14.48: Amniocentesis is:

a) a procedure for detecting fetal abnormalities
b) an infection of the brain
c) a condition affecting the sex chromosomes
d) an inability to metabolize phenylalanine

MC/Easy
Pg:492
kind:f
Ans:(a)

14.49: Research on the effectiveness of Head Start, an
intervention program for disadvantaged
preschoolers, has shown:

a) improved health but no differences in academic
performance
b) long-term increases in IQ levels
c) short-term increases in IQ and academic
achievement
d) no reduction in cultural-familial retardation

MC/Mod
Pg:492
kind:c
Ans:(c)

14.50: Although operant behavior therapy is an effective
means of controlling behavior problems among the
mentally retarded, many institutionalized patients
with mental retardation are prescribed neuroleptic
medication. This practice is controversial because
these drugs:

a) can be misused as sedatives
b) are addictive
c) can actually increase aggression
d) predispose patients to psychosis

MC/Mod
Pg:493
kind:c
Ans:(a)

14.51: Public Law 94-142, the "Education for All   MC/Mod
       Handicapped Children Act" (1975) was important   Pg:493
       because it introduced for the first time: kind:c
                                                            Ans:(d)
       a) special education classes
       b) inclusion of mental retardation in the category
          of "handicapped"
       c) treatment of emotional and behavioral problems
          by school personnel
       d) a requirement that all children be educated in
          the least restrictive environment

14.52: Compared to a mentally retarded person with an IQ   MC/Mod
       of 70, a person with pervasive developmental   Pg:494
       disorder and an IQ of 70 is likely to show more   kind:c
       problems in the area of: Ans:(c)

       a) physical development
       b) perceptual abilities
       c) relationships
       d) psychotic symptoms

14.53: Which of the following characterizes the physical   MC/Easy
       appearance of autistic children?   Pg:495
                                                            kind:f
       a) facial features have a "mongoloid" appearance   Ans:(c)
       b) retarded physical development and small head
          circumference
       c) normal physical appearance
       d) uncoordinated movements

14.54: Two of the classical symptoms of autism are   MC/Mod
       impaired social relationships and stereotyped   Pg:495
       behavior. The other classical symptoms of autism   kind:c
       is: Ans:(d)

       a) delayed physical development
       b) "mongoloid" facial features
       c) inability to metabolize phenylalanine
       d) impaired communication ability

14.55: Gaze-aversion in children with pervasive   MC/Mod
       developmental disorder and autism is thought to be Pg:495
       an indication of: kind:c
                                                            Ans:(c)
       a) motor coordination problems
       b) perceptual difficulties
       c) discomfort with social interactions
       d) hallucinations

14.56: Which of the following is a likely description of   MC/Mod
       how an autistic child might interact with his   Pg:495
       mother?   kind:a
                                                            Ans:(b)
       a) jealous and demanding of mother's attention
       b) doesn't like to be held
       c) cries a lot and wants comforting
       d) looks at mother a lot, trying to communicate
          with her nonverbally

14.57: The communication patterns of many autistic people MC/Mod
       are characterized by dysprosody. This is: Pg:496
                                                            kind:f
       a) meaningless repetition of phrases   Ans:(c)
       b) pronoun reversal
       c) abnormal rate, rhythm, and intonation of speech
       d) bizarre content of speech

14.58: Which of the following is a common language problem MC/Easy
       among autistic children?   Pg:497
                                                            kind:f
       a) rambling and meaningless stories   Ans:(c)
       b) poor articulation due to deafness
       c) using "you" instead of "I"
       d) preference for gestures rather than verbal
          language

14.59: Communication difficulties and impaired social   MC/Mod
       relationships in autistic children are thought to   Pg:497
       have in common a more basic problem of: kind:c
                                                            Ans:(b)
       a) perceptual impairment
       b) lack of social imitation and reciprocity
       c) motor impairments
       d) psychotic disturbances

14.60: One of the major symptoms of autism and other pervasive developmental disorders is behavior that is:

    a) manipulative and antisocial
    b) dependent and emotionally needy
    c) psychotic in nature
    d) restrictive and repetitive

MC/Easy
Pg:497
kind:f
Ans:(d)

14.61: Which of the following is an example of the "apparent sensory deficits" seen in some autistic children?

    a) unusual response to certain sounds
    b) lack of sensory input and need for self-stimulation
    c) mutism due to deafness
    d) gaze aversion because of visual impairments

MC/Mod
Pg:498
kind:c
Ans:(a)

14.62: On rare occasions, a person with autism or another pervasive developmental disorder shows savant performance. This is:

    a) an exceptional skill in a very specific area
    b) very high IQ and superior intelligence
    c) self-stimulatory behavior
    d) self-injurious behavior

MC/Mod
Pg:498
kind:c
Ans:(a)

14.63: Which of the following is a typical area of savant performance?

    a) linguistics   b) athletics
    c) creative writing   d) mathematics

MC/Easy
Pg:498
kind:f
Ans:(d)

14.64: Early descriptions of the core behaviors of autism were made by:

    a) Down   b) Kanner
    c) Klinefelter   d) Turner

MC/Easy
Pg:498
kind:f
Ans:(b)

14.65: Asperger's disorder is descriptively identical to   MC/Mod
autism, except that in Asperger's disorder, there   Pg:499
is: kind:c
                                                             Ans:(a)

    a) higher intelligence and no language delay
    b) accompanying physical impairment
    c) more severe disturbances in relationships
    d) less stereotypical behavior

14.66: The onset of autistic-like disturbances in social   MC/Mod
interaction and communication after the age of 2 is   Pg:499
part of a condition called: kind:c
                                                             Ans:(a)

    a) childhood disintegrative disorder
    b) Rett's disorder
    c) Asperger's disorder
    d) childhood schizophrenia

14.67: A form of pervasive developmental disorder that   MC/Mod
involves language and social impairment,   Pg:499
deceleration of head growth, and poor coordination   kind:c
after a period of normal development is: Ans:(a)

    a) Rett's disorder
    b) childhood disintegrative disorder
    c) Asperger's disorder
    d) childhood schizophrenia

14.68: Compared to pervasive developmental disorder,   MC/Diff
mental retardation and aphasia show: Pg:499
                                                             kind:c
    a) less use of gestures to communicate   Ans:(b)
    b) more sociability
    c) more motor and physical impairments
    d) lower intelligence

14.69: The highly unusual ability to recite the day of the   MC/Easy
week for any date is an example of a rare   Pg:500
characteristic of autism called: kind:c
                                                             Ans:(b)

    a) dysprosody
    b) savant performance
    c) Asperger's syndrome
    d) apparent sensory deficit

281

14.70: Autism is more common in:

    a) higher classes   b) lower classes
    c) girls   d) boys

MC/Mod
Pg:501
kind:f
Ans:(d)

14.71: Research has shown that parents of autistic children:

    a) are cold and distant
    b) are abusive
    c) are usually highly intelligent and of the upper class
    d) have similar child rearing styles as other parents

MC/Mod
Pg:501
kind:c
Ans:(d)

14.72: In scientific research the null hypothesis is:

    a) a new idea that has yet to be proven
    b) an easily dismissed, absurd notion
    c) an idea that has been shown to be false
    d) an idea that is assumed to be true until proven false

MC/Mod
Pg:502
kind:c
Ans:(d)

14.73: Which of the following is true about the biological factors involved in autism?

    a) many autistic persons have genetic and neurological abnormalities
    b) autism does not run in families
    c) very few autistic persons show seizure disorders
    d) Down syndrome is especially common in autistic persons

MC/Mod
Pg:503
kind:c
Ans:(a)

14.74: The risk of autism among siblings of autistic patients is:

    a) the same as that of the general population
    b) 50 times higher than in the general population
    c) twice as high as in the general population
    d) lower than in the general population

MC/Easy
Pg:503
kind:f
Ans:(b)

14.75: There is preliminary evidence that fenfluramine may   MC/Mod
alleviate some symptoms of autism by: Pg:504
    kind:c

    a) reducing serotonin levels   Ans:(a)
    b) increasing serotonin levels
    c) reducing dopamine levels
    d) increasing dopamine levels

14.76: The type of structural brain abnormality associated   MC/Mod
with autism is thought to be due to: Pg:505
    kind:c

    a) specific damage to a formerly normal brain   Ans:(c)
    b) lesions
    c) abnormalities in early brain development
    d) plasticity

14.77: Which of the following describes the course of   MC/Easy
autism?   Pg:505
    kind:f

    a) often resolves itself by age 5 or 6   Ans:(d)
    b) often resolves itself at puberty
    c) often resolves itself in young adulthood
    d) a lifelong disorder

14.78: The cognitive and social skills of autistic   MC/Mod
children often show a noticeable turn for the worse   Pg:505
or better at what developmental period?   kind:f
    Ans:(b)

    a) preschool   b) early adolescence
    c) young adulthood   d) middle age

14.79: "Facilitated communication" is a controversial   MC/Easy
technique in which persons with communication   Pg:506
disorders are helped to communicate by: kind:f
    Ans:(a)

    a) typing while another person supports their arm
    b) glancing at pictures on a computer
    c) pointing to pictures on a card
    d) using American Sign Language

14.80: "Facilitated communication" is a technique whereby persons with communication disorders type with the help of an assistant. One reason that the use of this technique with autistics has been called into question is that:

    a) these patients are unable to learn how to type
    b) autistics lack the motor coordination to type
    c) the assistant's presence affects the patients' responses
    d) autistic patients do not like to be touched

MC/Mod
Pg:506
kind:c
Ans:(c)

14.81: Psychodynamic therapies to treat autism, now for the most part abandoned, attempted to:

    a) flood the child with exposure to other children
    b) use hypnotism to uncover childhood trauma
    c) encourage less involvement by doting parents
    d) foster attachment to the therapist

MC/Mod
Pg:508
kind:c
Ans:(d)

14.82: In behavior modification for specific behaviors associated with autism, which of the following would be the most effective reinforcer?

    a) a pat on the head or a hug
    b) the child's favorite food
    c) a smile and the comment "great!"
    d) getting to play a game with mother

MC/Diff
Pg:508
kind:c
Ans:(b)

14.83: Through behavior modification, autistic children can learn basic communication in a process that:

    a) is very similar to normal language learning
    b) is very different from normal language learning
    c) relies on sign language rather than verbal expression
    d) uses social interaction and praise as reinforcers

MC/Diff
Pg:508
kind:c
Ans:(b)

14.84: Behavior modification to extinguish self-injurious behaviors usually relies on a process of:

    a) punishment
    b) positive reinforcement
    c) negative reinforcement
    d) response cost

MC/Easy
Pg:508
kind:f
Ans:(a)

14.85: Lovaas has conducted research on autistic children who undergo several years of intensive behavior modification. This research shows that in these children, rates of completing 1st grade are:

    a) much higher than in control groups
    b) the same as in control groups
    c) unrelated to IQ
    d) unrelated to parenting styles

MC/Diff
Pg:509
kind:c
Ans:(a)

True-False Questions

14.86: Pervasive Developmental Disorder is a more common disorder than Mental Retardation.

TF/Easy
Pg:478
kind:f
Ans:False

14.87: Autism is the most severe form of Pervasive Developmental Disorder.

TF/Easy
Pg:478
kind:f
Ans:True

14.88: Most mentally retarded individuals are able to live in the community with little or no supervision.

TF/Easy
Pg:479
kind:f
Ans:True

14.89: IQ stands for "intelligence quotient."

TF/Easy
Pg:481
kind:f
Ans:True

14.90: An individually administered IQ test is required for a person to be diagnosed as mentally retarded.

TF/Easy
Pg:481
kind:f
Ans:True

14.91: The American Association on Mental Retardation (AAMR) describes mental retardation in terms of 4 levels of intensity of needed support.

TF/Mod
Pg:484
kind:c
Ans:True

14.92: Mildly mentally retarded persons typically have obvious physical abnormalities and impairments.

TF/Mod
Pg:484
kind:c
Ans:False

14.93: Only males can inherit fragile X syndrome.

TF/Mod
Pg:486
kind:f
Ans:False

14.94: Children with PKU are born with normal intelligence but develop brain damage and mental retardation over time.

TF/Mod
Pg:487
kind:f
Ans:True

14.95: A stimulating environment and access to more educational resources can increase the IQ of a person with mild mental retardation.

TF/Mod
Pg:491
kind:f
Ans:True

14.96: Many cases of mental retardation are not detected in preschoolers because IQ tests are unreliable in this age group.

TF/Mod
Pg:492
kind:c
Ans:True

14.97: For many mentally retarded children, education in the "least restrictive environment" means mainstreaming in a regular classroom.

TF/Mod
Pg:493
kind:c
Ans:True

14.98: Most people with pervasive developmental disorder are also mentally retarded.

TF/Mod
Pg:494
kind:f
Ans:True

14.99: Autistic children who are mute often use gestures as substitutes for speech.

TF/Mod
Pg:497
kind:f
Ans:False

14.100: Most people with autism learn how to communicate using sign language.

TF/Mod
Pg:497
kind:f
Ans:False

14.101: The self-injurious behavior shown by some autistics is a form of suicidal behavior.

TF/Mod
Pg:498
kind:f
Ans:False

14.102: Autism is more common among those in higher socioeconomic groups.

TF/Easy
Pg:501
kind:f
Ans:False

14.103: The siblings of autistic children are at greater risk for autism than is the general population.

TF/Easy
Pg:501
kind:f
Ans:True

14.104: A researcher believes that autism is caused by poor nutrition. If this is the experimental hypothesis, the null hypothesis is that autism is NOT caused by poor nutrition.

TF/Diff
Pg:502
kind:a
Ans:True

Essay Questions

14.105: Describe the controversy around the issue of whether IQ tests are "culture fair."

Answer: On average, the IQ scores of African-Americans and Latino-Americans are lower than those of Caucasians and Asian-Americans, and the rates of mental retardation are also higher in these former groups. Some of these differences have been attributed to bias in the composition of intelligence tests, which may be geared toward the majority group. It is for this reason that the AAMR requires valid assessment that considers cultural and linguistic diversity.

ES Moderate Pages: 481-482 kind: c

14.106: What are the 2 aspects of adaptive skills that are evaluated in making the diagnosis of mental retardation? Give an example of each.

Answer: Practical intelligence, such as cooking and brushing one's teeth; social intelligence, such as asking someone for help and greeting someone at the door.

ES Moderate Page: 482 kind: c

14.107: At different points in time, the American Association of Mental Retardation (AAMR) has used different IQ cutoff points, including 70, 85, and 70-75. Why were these cutoffs chosen? Why were earlier cutoffs abandoned?

Answer: 70 was chosen because it is equivalent to 2 standard deviations below the mean, an accepted definition of mental retardation based on statistical rarity. 85 was chosen because it is only 1 standard deviation below the mean; with this score, there is a better chance of correctly identifying all mentally retarded individuals, but there is also a higher chance of including too many well-functioning individuals, as this cutoff included 15% of the population. The cutoff range of 70-75 is currently being used because it takes into account measurement error and recognizes that a score of 69 is not statistically different from a score of 71.

ES   Moderate   Pages: 483-484   kind: c

14.108: Although more than 3% of the population have IQs below 70, only about 1% of people are diagnosed as mentally retarded at any one point in time. Explain the reasons for this discrepancy.

Answer: Many young children who are mentally retarded are not identified as such because it is difficult to obtain a reliable IQ score from people this age. Also, many adults who have IQs under 70 function adaptively, and so are not considered mentally retarded.

ES   Moderate   Page: 485   kind: c

14.109: Describe the concept of a reaction range and how it relates to intelligence level.

Answer: Genes and environment interact to produce intelligence. The concept of a reaction range holds that heredity establishes the upper and lower limits of possible IQ, but experience determines the extent to which a person fulfills his or her potential.

ES   Moderate   Page: 490   kind: c

14.110: Describe the 2 alternative interpretations of "self-stimulating" behaviors seen in autistics, such as hand flapping and watching a top spin.

Answer: The child could be self-stimulating because he or she receives too little sensory input; alternatively, the child could be overwhelmed and is trying to reduce input by focusing on a monotonous, predictable stimulus.

ES   Moderate   Page: 497   kind: c

14.111: Explain why the term "childhood schizophrenia" is an inappropriate label for autism.

Answer: The symptoms of autism and schizophrenia are very different, and the two disorders remain different over time. The symptoms of autism manifest themselves in early childhood, whereas the symptoms of schizophrenia are not present until adolescence.

ES   Moderate   Page: 499   kind: c

Chapter 15
Psychological Problems of Childhood
and Eating Disorders

Multiple Choice Questions

15.1: An example of an externalizing disorder is: MC/Easy
Pg:514

    a) anxiety   b) depression   kind:c
    c) conduct disorder   d) somatization   Ans:(c)

15.2: The most commonly diagnosed psychological problems MC/Mod
in children are: Pg:514

                                               kind:f
    a) eating disorders   Ans:(c)
    b) internalizing disorders
    c) externalizing disorders
    d) developmental disorders

15.3: An example of an internalizing disorder is: MC/Easy
Pg:514

    a) depression   kind:c
    b) attention deficit/hyperactivity disorder Ans:(a)
    c) oppositional defiant disorder
    d) conduct disorder

15.4: The major contribution of a developmental MC/Easy
psychopathology perspective on children's problems Pg:515
is that it takes into account: kind:c

                                               Ans:(d)
    a) biological processes
    b) environmental differences across socioeconomic
       groups
    c) genetics
    d) norms across the lifespan

15.5: Externalizing disorders are characterized by: MC/Easy
Pg:517

    a) expression of worry through physical symptoms kind:c
    b) symptoms of sadness and anxiety   Ans:(d)
    c) overcontrolled behavior
    d) violations of age-appropriate social rules

15.6: Evidence for a syndrome of externalizing behavior problems has been demonstrated by statistical analysis of:

    a) children's descriptions of their own behavior
    b) checklists on which adults rate children's problems
    c) clinicians' diagnoses of children
    d) arrest reports

MC/Diff
Pg:518
kind:c
Ans:(b)

15.7: About what percentage of arrests for index offenses (such as murder, rape, robbery) are of juveniles younger than 18?

    a) 1%   b) 10%
    c) 30%   d) 50%

MC/Mod
Pg:518
kind:f
Ans:(c)

15.8: It is developmentally normal for children to begin to test limits and to resist rules beginning at about age:

    a) 6 months   b) 1 year
    c) 2 years   d) 4 years

MC/Mod
Pg:519
kind:f
Ans:(c)

15.9: The ultimate goal of socialization is:

    a) conformity to external influences
    b) internal, self-control of behavior
    c) secure attachment to a parental figure
    d) psychological health

MC/Easy
Pg:519
kind:c
Ans:(b)

15.10: The best predictor of adult antisocial behavior is:

    a) antisocial behavior in adolescence
    b) withdrawn behavior in adolescence
    c) antisocial behavior in childhood
    d) withdrawn behavior in childhood

MC/Mod
Pg:519
kind:c
Ans:(c)

15.11: Chris begins to show externalizing and antisocial behaviors at age 6. Doug begins to show these behaviors at age 16. Compared to Doug, Chris's problems:

MC/Mod
Pg:519
kind:a
Ans:(d)

a) will probably have a shorter duration
b) are probably less disruptive to other people
c) will be more related to health problems
d) have a higher chance of persisting throughout life

15.12: An example of an internalizing symptom is:

MC/Easy
Pg:520
kind:c
Ans:(a)

a) sadness   b) fighting
c) hyperactivity   d) talking back

15.13: The criteria for the diagnoses of phobia and depression in children are slightly different from those used to diagnose these disorders in adults. The criteria for children take into account children's:

MC/Mod
Pg:520
kind:c
Ans:(d)

a) different physiological symptoms
b) more frequent suicidal ideation
c) different responsiveness to medications
d) limited cognitive capacity for insight

15.14: Which of the following describes ratings made by parents and children concerning children's internalizing problems?

MC/Mod
Pg:520
kind:c
Ans:(b)

a) parents overestimate children's depression
b) parents underestimate children's depression
c) parents' and children's ratings of severity are highly correlated
d) parents' and children's ratings of symptoms are highly correlated

15.15: Which of the following characterizes the development of children's fears?

MC/Mod
Pg:521
kind:c
Ans:(b)

a) frequency of fears increases with age
b) different fears develop for the first time at different ages
c) fears are a sign of pathology
d) 8-year-olds and 16-year-olds have no fears in common

15.16: A common fear that is prevalent from ages 8 through 16 is:

a) not being able to breathe
b) the dark
c) separation from parents
d) being humiliated in public

MC/Diff
Pg:521
kind:f
Ans:(a)

15.17: Fears that are common in children of all ages appear to focus on:

a) being humiliated by others in public
b) uncontrollable events such as accidents and war
c) being physically attacked by peers
d) losing material possessions

MC/Mod
Pg:521
kind:c
Ans:(b)

15.18: Separation anxiety, or the fear of separation from caretakers, is a normal fear that typically develops around age:

a) 6 months   b) 1 year
c) 2 years   d) 3 years

MC/Mod
Pg:521
kind:f
Ans:(b)

15.19: In a 1-year-old child, separation anxiety, or distress at being separated from one's caretakers, is:

a) a normal fear
b) a sign of pathology
c) highly unusual
d) not upsetting for the child

MC/Mod
Pg:521
kind:c
Ans:(a)

15.20: School phobia, or the refusal to go to school, is often associated with:

a) anger at parents
b) anger at teachers
c) separation anxiety disorder
d) externalizing disorders

MC/Mod
Pg:521
kind:c
Ans:(c)

15.21: One disruptive consequence of separation anxiety disorder is:

a) fighting with peers   b) delinquency
c) school refusal   d) hyperactivity

MC/Easy
Pg:522
kind:c
Ans:(c)

15.22: The peer sociometric method involves:

    a) children's ratings of their peers' popularity
    b) teachers' ratings of children's friendships
    c) sociologists' observations of children's alliances
    d) training for children on how to make friends

MC/Mod
Pg:523
kind:c
Ans:(a)

15.23: Sociometric methods allow the classification of children as popular, average, neglected, rejected, and controversial. Which of these categories show the highest rates of internalizing disorders?

    a) neglected   b) rejected
    c) average   d) controversial

MC/Diff
Pg:523
kind:c
Ans:(a)

15.24: Parents' ratings of their children's externalizing problems are sometimes worse than clinicians' observations of the same problems. Part of this discrepancy may be due to reactivity. Reactivity refers to:

    a) parents' sensitivity to their children's problems
    b) changes in child behavior when observed
    c) clinicians' high threshold for identifying problems
    d) different results based on which checklist is used

MC/Mod
Pg:523
kind:c
Ans:(b)

15.25: Although antisocial behavior and depression in childhood often continue to be problems in adulthood, the problems in adulthood are not isomorphic with those in childhood. This means that in the adult form:

    a) the disorder is more severe
    b) the disorder is less severe
    c) the disorder has very different causes
    d) the disorder is the same, but expressed differently

MC/Mod
Pg:524
kind:c
Ans:(d)

15.26: A rare disorder involving the persistent eating of non-nutritive substances such as paint and dirt is:

    a) rumination disorder   b) encopresis
    c) pica   d) Tourette's disorder

MC/Mod
Pg:524
kind:f
Ans:(c)

15.27: Tourette's disorder is a rare problem characterized by:

    a) motor and verbal tics
    b) eating of non-nutritive substances
    c) uncontrolled urination
    d) regurgitation and rechewing of food

MC/Mod
Pg:525
kind:f
Ans:(a)

15.28: A disorder thought to result from a failure to develop a selective attachment relationship is called:

    a) Tourette's disorder
    b) reactive attachment disorder
    c) separation anxiety disorder
    d) oppositional defiant disorder

MC/Mod
Pg:525
kind:f
Ans:(b)

15.29: Bedwetting is a symptom of:

    a) pica   b) rumination
    c) encopresis   d) enuresis

MC/Easy
Pg:525
kind:f
Ans:(d)

15.30: The bell and pad device is used to treat:

    a) pica   b) Tourette's disorder
    c) enuresis   d) selective mutism

MC/Easy
Pg:525
kind:f
Ans:(c)

15.31: DSM-IV's section on disorders of childhood has been criticized for including:

    a) too few disorders affecting children
    b) too many internalizing categories
    c) too few externalizing categories
    d) too many non-psychiatric disorders

MC/Diff
Pg:526
kind:c
Ans:(d)

15.32: Jose is given an IQ test and an academic achievement test. Based on which test results might he be classified as having a learning disability?

    a) IQ less than 70
    b) achievement score 2 grades behind normal
    c) average achievement test scores, but unusual
       learning style
    d) IQ score significantly higher than achievement
       test score

MC/Mod
Pg:526
kind:a
Ans:(d)

15.33: Which of the following describes DSM-IV's inclusion of childhood internalizing disorders?

    a) the first time any internalizing disorders were included
    b) none included, despite empirical evidence
    c) none included, based on empirical evidence
    d) too many included

MC/Mod
Pg:527
kind:c
Ans:(b)

15.34: In the 1800s, children with externalizing disorders were seen as having weak moral characters. In the early 1900s, what is now called attention deficit/hyperactivity disorder came to be viewed not as a moral failing but as a result of:

    a) ineffective parenting
    b) failures of the educational system
    c) minimal brain damage
    d) anxiety

MC/Mod
Pg:527
kind:c
Ans:(c)

15.35: Psychostimulant medications that are used to increase energy and alertness reduce hyperactivity in children with attention deficit/hyperactivity disorder. In normal children, these drugs:

    a) have the same effect
    b) produce increased hyperactivity
    c) have no effect
    d) reduce alertness

MC/Mod
Pg:528
kind:c
Ans:(a)

15.36: Compared to conduct disorder, oppositional-defiant disorder tends to:

    a) involve more serious rule violation
    b) occur in older children
    c) occur in younger children
    d) be more closely associated with minimal brain damage

MC/Mod
Pg:528
kind:c
Ans:(c)

15.37: Some of the diagnostic criteria for conduct disorder are comparable to status offenses. Status offenses are:

    a) crimes that are illegal at any age
    b) acts that are illegal only if you are a minor
    c) behaviors that are disruptive but not illegal
    d) behaviors that are legal but morally questionable

MC/Mod
Pg:529
kind:c
Ans:(b)

15.38: Hyperactivity is most notable in:

    a) structured situations such as the classroom
    b) unstructured situations such as the playground
    c) unfamiliar places
    d) the physician's office

MC/Mod
Pg:529
kind:c
Ans:(a)

15.39: Attention deficit/hyperactivity disorder is typically first diagnosed:

    a) at age 2-3
    b) in the early school years
    c) in early adolescence
    d) in late adolescence

MC/Mod
Pg:529
kind:f
Ans:(b)

15.40: According to the National Academy of Sciences, about what percentage of children in the U.S. have a mental disorder?

    a) 1%   b) 3%
    c) 6%   d) 12%

MC/Easy
Pg:531
kind:f
Ans:(d)

15.41: In order for research results to be generalizable, a researcher needs:

    a) a small convenience sample
    b) data on the whole population of interest
    c) a large representative sample
    d) information from interviews and other "global" measures

MC/Mod
Pg:532
kind:c
Ans:(c)

15.42: Which of the following characterizes the association between gender and externalizing disorders?

    a) more common in girls
    b) more common in boys
    c) in both genders, increase with age
    d) equally prevalent among men and women

MC/Mod
Pg:533
kind:c
Ans:(b)

15.43: Since the 1960s, suicide rates have tripled among which age group?

    a) age 10-14   b) adolescents
    c) young adults   d) elderly

MC/Easy
Pg:534
kind:f
Ans:(b)

15.44: In comparison to adult suicide attempts, suicide
attempts by adolescents are:

    a) less impulsive
    b) more motivated by depression than anger
    c) less likely to require therapy
    d) more likely to follow family conflict

MC/Mod
Pg:534
kind:f
Ans:(d)

15.45: Rutter studied the association between
externalizing disorders and family adversity,
including low income, overcrowded living
conditions, and family conflict. Which of the
following typifies this association?

    a) no association between family problems and
       externalizing disorders
    b) presence of 1 adversity factor associated with
       much higher externalizing
    c) presence of 2 adversity factors associated with
       much higher externalizing
    d) no externalizing problems if no family problems

MC/Mod
Pg:534
kind:c
Ans:(c)

15.46: Bowlby, Ainsworth, and colleagues proposed that
psychopathology is caused by:

    a) troubled attachments
    b) genetic predisposition
    c) biochemical imbalance
    d) children's imitation of parent problems

MC/Easy
Pg:535
kind:f
Ans:(a)

15.47: Nonhuman primates who are raised in isolation
without a parent or substitute attachment figure:

    a) have dramatically troubled relationships
    b) develop normal socially
    c) show problems until adolescence
    d) show no problems until adolescence

MC/Mod
Pg:535
kind:c
Ans:(a)

15.48: In the case of anxious attachment:

    a) the child experiences anxiety about exploration
    b) no selective attachment is formed
    c) the parent responds consistently to the child
    d) the child experiences anaclitic depression

MC/Mod
Pg:535
kind:c
Ans:(a)

15.49: After the loss of an attachment figure, children go through stages of reaction akin to grief, the last stage being:

MC/Mod
Pg:535
kind:c
Ans:(b)

a) numbness
c) protest

b) detachment
d) despair

15.50: The most effective parenting style is:

MC/Easy
Pg:535
kind:c
Ans:(b)

a) indulgent
c) authoritarian

b) authoritative
d) secure

15.51: Which of the following describes authoritarian parenting?

MC/Easy
Pg:535
kind:c
Ans:(d)

a) loving and firm
b) affectionate but lax
c) unconcerned
d) strict and lacking warmth

15.52: Children with serious conduct problems often have parents who are:

MC/Mod
Pg:536
kind:f
Ans:(c)

a) authoritarian
c) neglectful

b) authoritative
d) indulgent

15.53: According to Patterson's social learning model of the development of externalizing disorders, coercion is best described as a process of:

MC/Mod
Pg:536
kind:c
Ans:(b)

a) manipulation by children
b) reciprocal influences between parents and children
c) control by parents
d) getting families to follow treatment recommendations

15.54: Patterson's social learning model holds that coercion is key to understanding the development of externalizing disorder. Coercion is a process of:

MC/Mod
Pg:536
kind:c
Ans:(c)

a) purposeful reinforcement for bad behavior
b) purposeful punishment for bad behavior
c) inadvertent reinforcement for bad behavior
d) inadvertent punishment for bad behavior

15.55: Brief isolation after misbehavior is called:

    a) coercion   b) negative attention
    c) detachment   d) time out

MC/Easy
Pg:536
kind:c
Ans:(d)

15.56: In general, children with externalizing disorders have been found to show:

    a) detachment
    b) anaclitic depression
    c) negative attention
    d) inability to delay gratification

MC/Mod
Pg:537
kind:c
Ans:(d)

15.57: Which of the following is true about aggressive children?

    a) show less advanced moral reasoning
    b) delay gratification for too long
    c) don't notice peers' aggressive intentions
    d) show detachment and lack attachment

MC/Mod
Pg:538
kind:c
Ans:(a)

15.58: Triple blind studies of medication effectiveness (where neither the physician nor the parent nor the child is aware of whether the medication is active or a placebo) show that the behavior of children with attention deficit/hyperactivity disorder improves on medication, and that mothers' behavior:

    a) is unaffected
    b) is less negative and less controlling
    c) is more negative and more controlling
    d) improves only if she guesses that the child is on medication

MC/Mod
Pg:538
kind:c
Ans:(b)

15.59: One factor that may be genetically mediated and that is thought to cause oppositional defiant disorder and conduct disorder is:

    a) chronic underarousal of the autonomic nervous system
    b) chronic overarousal of the autonomic nervous system
    c) chronic underarousal of the central nervous system
    d) chronic overarousal of the central nervous system

MC/Mod
Pg:539
kind:c
Ans:(a)

15.60: Which is true of the neurological problems associated with attention deficit/hyperactivity disorder?

MC/Mod
Pg:539
kind:c
Ans:(b)

a) hard signs such as abnormal CT scans are common
b) soft signs are more common than average
c) neurochemical differences are clear markers of vulnerability
d) impairment has been localized to the left hemisphere

15.61: The Feingold diet, a popular diet for children with attention deficit/hyperactivity disorder, purportedly decreased hyperactivity by:

MC/Easy
Pg:539
kind:f
Ans:(b)

a) eliminating sugar
b) eliminating food additives
c) supplementing diet with vitamin C
d) supplementing diet with phenylalanines

15.62: Research on the association between diet and attention deficit/hyperactivity disorder has shown:

MC/Mod
Pg:539
kind:c
Ans:(c)

a) sugar increases hyperactivity
b) food additives increase hyperactivity
c) there is no relationship between diet and hyperactivity
d) preservatives increase hyperactivity

15.63: Which is true about the overlap of attention deficit/hyperactivity disorder and oppositional-defiant disorder?

MC/Mod
Pg:540
kind:f
Ans:(d)

a) very little overlap
b) children diagnosed as oppositional almost always later show ADHD
c) children diagnosed as ADHD almost always later show oppositionality
d) about 50% of children with 1 disorder also have the other

15.64: Some researchers have suggested that socialized delinquency is a subtype of externalizing disorder. This subtype is characterized by:

a) formerly aggressive children later becoming obedient
b) criminal acts occurring in the company of others
c) "hidden" criminality such as "white collar" crime
d) delinquency learned from one's parents

MC/Mod
Pg:540
kind:c
Ans:(b)

15.65: The highest rates of homicide among males aged 15-24 are found in which country?

a) Ireland   b) U.S.
c) Israel   d) Colombia

MC/Easy
Pg:540
kind:f
Ans:(b)

15.66: About what percentage of all school children in the U.S. are treated with psychostimulant medication for attention deficit/hyperactivity disorder each year?

a) 0.5%   b) 1-2%
c) 5%   d) 10%

MC/Diff
Pg:541
kind:f
Ans:(b)

15.67: In about what percentage of children with attention deficit/hyperactivity disorder who are taking psychostimulant medication is there an immediate benefit of medication?

a) 10%   b) 25%
c) 50%   d) 75%

MC/Mod
Pg:541
kind:f
Ans:(d)

15.68: Children who take Ritalin, Dexedrine, and Cylert, psychostimulants used in the treatment of attention-deficit/hyperactivity disorder, typically do so for:

a) a few days   b) a few weeks
c) a few months   d) years

MC/Easy
Pg:542
kind:f
Ans:(d)

15.69: Which is true about the effect of psychostimulant medication on children's school performance?

MC/Mod
Pg:542
kind:f
Ans:(b)

    a) improved grades
    b) more accurate completion of assignments
    c) improved achievement test scores
    d) better scores in reading but not math

15.70: One of the most important side effects of psychostimulant medications is:

MC/Mod
Pg:542
kind:f
Ans:(c)

    a) depression
    b) nausea and vomiting
    c) slower gains in height and weight
    d) itching and rashes

15.71: A central process in behavioral family therapy to treat adolescents with conduct disorder is:

MC/Mod
Pg:543
kind:c
Ans:(d)

    a) helping the parents gain more control over the adolescent
    b) getting the parents to be less authoritative
    c) fostering empathic understanding rather than behavior management
    d) promoting adolescent's involvement in deciding the rules

15.72: Research on residential programs such as Achievement Place, a group home that operates on highly structured behavior therapy principles, shows:

MC/Mod
Pg:544
kind:f
Ans:(d)

    a) lower rates of recidivism once the teen leaves the program
    b) long-term reductions in aggression
    c) few results while the teen in still in the group home
    d) effective results while the teen is living in the group home

15.73: Anorexia nervosa is characterized by:

MC/Easy
Pg:544
kind:c
Ans:(d)

    a) repeated episodes of binge eating
    b) self-induced vomiting
    c) eating non-nutrient substances
    d) restricted eating and below-normal body weight

15.74: Bulimia nervosa is characterized by:

    a) very low body weight
    b) binge eating and purging
    c) amenorrhea
    d) eating non-nutritive substances

MC/Easy
Pg:544
kind:c
Ans:(b)

15.75: One psychological difference between bulimia nervosa and anorexia nervosa is that anorexia is characterized by:

    a) shame about lack of control
    b) lack of rituals around eating
    c) lack of anxiety
    d) pride in self-control

MC/Mod
Pg:545
kind:c
Ans:(d)

15.76: One diagnostic criterion of anorexia nervosa is amenorrhea. This is:

    a) less than 85% expected body weight
    b) absence of menstruation
    c) disturbed body image
    d) undue influence of body shape on self-evaluation

MC/Easy
Pg:546
kind:f
Ans:(b)

15.77: Which is true about the epidemiology of eating disorders?

    a) bulimia is more common than anorexia
    b) anorexia is more common than bulimia
    c) there is very little overlap between eating disorders
    d) eating disorders are less common now than in the past

MC/Mod
Pg:547
kind:f
Ans:(a)

15.78: Eating disorders are diagnosed about 10 times more frequently among females than among males. This discrepancy is thought to be due to:

    a) hormonal differences in male and female teens
    b) differences in male and female brain structures
    c) methodological problems in detecting eating disorders in men
    d) societal expectations for gender roles

MC/Easy
Pg:547
kind:c
Ans:(d)

15.79: In what areas of the world are eating disorders found?

MC/Mod
Pg:547
kind:f
Ans:(c)

    a) in nearly all societies
    b) only in the U.S. and Canada
    c) almost exclusively in North America, Western Europe, and Japan
    d) in cultures with small population growth

15.80: The typical age of onset of eating disorders is around age:

MC/Mod
Pg:548
kind:c
Ans:(c)

    a) 8   b) 11
    c) 17   d) 26

15.81: One of the family patterns thought to contribute to the development of eating disorders is:

MC/Mod
Pg:548
kind:c
Ans:(d)

    a) modeling of disturbed eating by mothers
    b) parents ignoring their daughter's physical development
    c) being raised by a single parent
    d) lower parental tolerance for child autonomy

15.82: A psychological problem that often co-occurs with bulimia is:

MC/Easy
Pg:549
kind:f
Ans:(d)

    a) antisocial personality disorder
    b) histrionic personality disorder
    c) gender identity disorder
    d) depression

15.83: The area of the brain which regulates routine biological functions including appetite, and which has been hypothesized to be related to eating disorders, is the:

MC/Mod
Pg:549
kind:f
Ans:(c)

    a) hippocampus   b) striatum
    c) hypothalamus   d) cerebellum

15.84: Structural family therapists see the central problem in anorexia nervosa to be parents':

MC/Mod
Pg:549
kind:c
Ans:(c)

    a) authoritative parenting
    b) modeling of problematic eating patterns
    c) interference with adolescent's autonomy
    d) neglect and disinterest in their child

15.85: Researchers at the University of Minnesota have found that the most effective treatment for bulimia is:

    a) group psychotherapy
    b) antidepressant medications
    c) antianxiety medications
    d) education about nutrition and health

MC/Mod
Pg:550
kind:c
Ans:(a)

15.86: Among patients with anorexia nervosa, about what percentage starve themselves to death?

    a) 1%   b) 5%
    c) 10%   d) 15%

MC/Mod
Pg:551
kind:f
Ans:(b)

True-False Questions

15.87: Children cannot qualify for the adult diagnoses of mood disorder and anxiety disorder.

TF/Easy
Pg:514
kind:f
Ans:False

15.88: Eating disorders typically develop during adolescence.

TF/Easy
Pg:514
kind:f
Ans:True

15.89: Research has identified separate, distinct causes for attention deficit/hyperactivity disorder and conduct disorder.

TF/Mod
Pg:517
kind:c
Ans:False

15.90: Socialization is a process of shaping children's behavior to conform to societal expectations.

TF/Mod
Pg:518
kind:c
Ans:True

15.91: The major task of life during the first year is socialization.

TF/Easy
Pg:519
kind:c
Ans:False

15.92: Temper tantrums in a 2-year-old are a sign of psychological abnormality.

TF/Easy
Pg:519
kind:f
Ans:False

15.93: Separation anxiety is an externalizing disorder.

TF/Easy
Pg:521
kind:f
Ans:False

15.94: Often, school phobia is actually a fear of separation from one's caregiver.

TF/Easy
Pg:522
kind:c
Ans:True

15.95: The symptoms of depression in childhood are isomorphic to those in adulthood.

TF/Mod
Pg:524
kind:c
Ans:False

15.96: Children with learning disabilities rarely have attention deficit/hyperactivity disorder.

TF/Mod
Pg:526
kind:f
Ans:False

15.97: Juvenile delinquency is a term that refers to legal difficulties due to behaviors associated with conduct disorder.

TF/Easy
Pg:528
kind:f
Ans:True

15.98: Children with attention deficit/hyperactivity disorder typically show problems in immediate attention but no problems with sustained attention.

TF/Mod
Pg:530
kind:f
Ans:False

15.99: Cluster suicides are more common among teenagers than adults.

TF/Easy
Pg:534
kind:f
Ans:True

15.100: There is a greater genetic influence on adolescent-limited antisocial behavior than on life-course-persistent antisocial behavior.

TF/Mod
Pg:539
kind:f
Ans:False

307

15.101: The same drugs that help obsessive-compulsive disorder in adults help obsessive-compulsive disorder in children.

TF/Diff
Pg:541
kind:f
Ans:True

15.102: More treatments have been designed for externalizing disorders than internalizing disorders in children.

TF/Mod
Pg:541
kind:f
Ans:True

15.103: Ritalin, Dexedrine, and Cylert are sedatives used to treat attention-deficit disorder.

TF/Easy
Pg:541
kind:f
Ans:False

15.104: Children with attention deficit/hyperactivity disorder outgrow their inattention, hyperactivity, and impulsivity as adults.

TF/Mod
Pg:542
kind:f
Ans:False

15.105: Behavioral family therapy is more effective than medication in treating attention deficit/ hyperactivity disorder.

TF/Mod
Pg:543
kind:f
Ans:False

15.106: According to the diagnostic criteria of DSM-IV, purging in bulimia nervosa involves self-induced vomiting, but not other behaviors such as intense exercise or the use of laxatives.

TF/Mod
Pg:545
kind:f
Ans:False

15.107: Eating disorders are much more common now than they were in former centuries.

TF/Easy
Pg:546
kind:f
Ans:True

15.108: Treatment is easier and shows better outcomes with bulimia than anorexia.

TF/Mod
Pg:550
kind:f
Ans:True

Essay Questions

15.109: What special problems are associated with the assessment and diagnosis of children's psychological problems?

Answer: Children are often referred by an adult, whose report may be biased. In addition, it is difficult to assess children's inner states, as they have limited abilities for insight and verbal expression.

ES Moderate Page: 515 kind: c

15.110: Describe the societal changes in the 19th century that influenced the recognition of and attention to psychological problems in children.

Answer: Witmer established the first psychological clinic for children in the 19th century. Societal attitudes were also changing, with new emphasis on labor laws, mandatory schooling, and special juvenile courts. Childhood came to be seen as a stage characterized by the need for protection and nurturing.

ES Moderate Page: 524 kind: c

15.111: Explain the "paradoxical effect" of psychostimulant medication on children with attention deficit/hyperactivity disorder. How was this supposed effect used as evidence for minimal brain damage? How has this idea been shown to be erroneous?

Answer: Psychostimulant medications were found to "speed up" adults but slow down hyperactive children. This unexpected effect in children was taken as evidence of underlying brain abnormalities known as minimal brain damage. Later evidence showed, however, that normal children without attention deficit/hyperactivity disorder are also slowed down by these medications.

ES Moderate Page: 528 kind: c

15.112: Mental health professionals sometimes use convenience samples of patients who have presented for treatment. Give an example of when this would not be a methodological problem, and when it would be a methodological problem.

Answer: The use of convenience samples is not a problem in studies where the convenience sample is the same as the population of interest, such as studies of the effectiveness of medication or therapy techniques for people in therapy. Such samples are problematic, however, when conclusions about causality are drawn and generalizations are made to larger populations.

ES   Moderate   Pages: 531-532   kind: c

15.113: What are some of the reasons that more boys are treated for psychological problems than are girls, but more women are treated in therapy than are men?

Answer: Externalizing problems are more common in boys; these problems are more noticeable as a problem. The prevalence of externalizing behaviors decreases with age, whereas the prevalence of internalizing disorders increases with age. By adulthood, internalizing disorders (typically in women) are more common.

ES   Moderate   Page: 533   kind: c

15.114: According to attachment theorists, what problems in attachment are associated with psychopathology?

Answer: No selective attachment, insecure attachment, and multiple and prolonged separations from the caregiver.

ES   Moderate   Page: 535   kind: c

15.115: Explain the principle of parens patriae. What research evidence suggests that this principle may not be effectively practiced?

Answer: The state is to act as a parent for juveniles. Special juvenile courts are designed to guide, not punish, youth. However, data suggest that diversion out of the juvenile court system is more helpful than going through the court system.

ES   Moderate   Page: 544   kind: c

15.116: Explain why bulimia nervosa and anorexia nervosa are both considered to be characterized by a struggle for control.

Answer: People with bulimia feel out of control and ashamed of their lack of control, and their disorder is an attempt to regain a sense of control. People with anorexia pride themselves in self-control and their disorder is typified by excessive self-control.

ES   Moderate   Page: 545   kind: c

15.117: What patterns in the epidemiology of eating disorders suggest sociocultural influences on their development?

Answer: The prevalence of eating disorders is higher in industrialized societies such as North America, Western Europe, and Japan. In the U.S., the prevalence is higher in whites than blacks, those in higher SES groups, and women in jobs where slimness is valued. Eating disorders are also more frequent among groups who move into new areas where eating disorders exist, such as among Arabs and Asians who move to Europe and North America. Finally, in the U.S., there is an increasing number of eating disorder cases among middle class blacks.

ES   Moderate   Page: 548   kind: c

Chapter 16
Life Cycle Transitions and Adult Development

Multiple Choice Questions

16.1: Which of the following typifies life cycle transitions?

    a) they are mental disorders
    b) they occur in a predictable sequence
    c) they occur throughout adult development
    d) they involve little conflict

MC/Easy
Pg:556
kind:c
Ans:(c)

16.2: Adult development is characterized by:

    a) a sequence of time-limited stages
    b) a series of qualitatively different stages
    c) coping with a set of developmental tasks and challenges
    d) very little change or growth

MC/Mod
Pg:556
kind:c
Ans:(c)

16.3: Life cycle transitions are important to clinical psychologists because:

    a) they are a form of mental disorder
    b) many people seek help during a transition
    c) very few people experience them
    d) their timing and sequence indicate abnormality

MC/Easy
Pg:556
kind:f
Ans:(b)

16.4: Psychological problems can be conceptualized as residing in the individual, or as residing in the context of human relationships. How are these latter "interpersonal" diagnoses handled in DSM?

    a) first appeared in earlier versions of DSM
    b) first appeared in DSM-IV
    c) will probably be more common in future versions of DSM
    d) listed under personality disorders

MC/Easy
Pg:557
kind:f
Ans:(c)

16.5: Which of the following characterizes Erikson's
conceptualization of human development?

    a) healthy people experience little conflict
       during adult development
    b) psychosocial development is finished by young
       adulthood
    c) each stage involves a tension between
       stagnation and growth
    d) role confusion and identity are resolved by age
       5

MC/Mod
Pg:558
kind:c
Ans:(c)

16.6: Erikson viewed the primary life task of adolescence
to be a struggle between:

    a) role confusion and identity
    b) intimacy and self-absorption
    c) generativity and stagnation
    d) integrity and despair

MC/Mod
Pg:558
kind:c
Ans:(a)

16.7: Erikson viewed the primary life task of young
adulthood to be a struggle between:

    a) role confusion and identity
    b) intimacy and self-absorption
    c) integrity and despair
    d) generativity and stagnation

MC/Mod
Pg:558
kind:c
Ans:(b)

16.8: According to Erikson, generativity vs. stagnation
is a struggle inherent to which stage of adult
development?

    a) adolescence   b) young adulthood
    c) middle age   d) old age

MC/Mod
Pg:558
kind:c
Ans:(c)

16.9: In the DSM-IV, the "V-codes" are:

    a) on the 5th axis
    b) personality disorders
    c) disorders of old age
    d) conditions other than mental disorders that are
       the focus of treatment

MC/Easy
Pg:559
kind:f
Ans:(d)

16.10: How are life cycle transitions handled in the DSM-IV?

    a) listed as other conditions that may be the focus of treatment
    b) listed as causes of depression
    c) listed as a category of mental disorders
    d) listed under "relationship problems"

MC/Easy
Pg:559
kind:f
Ans:(a)

16.11: According to Erikson, the resolution of the identity crisis typically occurs in what developmental stage?

    a) childhood   b) adolescence
    c) middle age   d) old age

MC/Mod
Pg:559
kind:c
Ans:(b)

16.12: Erik Erikson's model of psychosocial development covered which age span?

    a) birth through age 5
    b) birth through age 12
    c) birth through adolescence
    d) birth through death

MC/Easy
Pg:559
kind:f
Ans:(d)

16.13: According to Erikson, the healthy resolution of the last stage of psychosocial development involves:

    a) pride in accomplishments and self-acceptance
    b) coherent sense of identity
    c) career achievements and a sense of direction
    d) balance between closeness and independence

MC/Mod
Pg:560
kind:c
Ans:(a)

16.14: According to Levinson's social model of adult development, the "midlife crisis" involves:

    a) becoming less driven and more compassionate
    b) moving away from family and assuming an adult role
    c) conflict between generativity and stagnation
    c) conflict between intimacy and self-absorption

MC/Diff
Pg:560
kind:c
Ans:(a)

16.15: One way that family life cycle theorists' view of adult development differs from Erikson's view of adult development is that in the family life cycle perspective there is:

MC/Mod
Pg:560
kind:c
Ans:(b)

a) greater focus on psychological changes within the individual
b) a definition of stages by addition and loss of family members
c) greater focus on the midlife crisis
d) less focus on intimacy

16.16: Erikson believed that a period of moratorium is necessary for adolescents to make a healthy transition to adulthood. By this he meant a period of:

MC/Mod
Pg:561
kind:c
Ans:(a)

a) uncertainty and experimentation with different roles
b) intimacy with a sexual partner
c) hard work and financial independence
d) balance between independence and closeness with parents

16.17: According to Erikson, teens need to experiment with different roles so that they can:

MC/Mod
Pg:562
kind:c
Ans:(d)

a) ease the separation from their parents
b) avoid moratorium
c) distract parents from their own conflicts
d) find a unique niche in society

16.18: During adolescence, a sense of certainty about personal identity is correlated with:

MC/Mod
Pg:562
kind:c
Ans:(b)

a) less intimacy with peers
b) less conflict with peers
c) more conflict with peers
d) more dependency on parents

16.19: The idea that relationship difficulties are due to conflicts among the needs to move toward, move away from and move against others was proposed by:

MC/Mod
Pg:562
kind:f
Ans:(a)

a) Horney
b) Bowlby
c) Erikson
d) Levinson

315

16.20: According to ego psychologist Karen Horney, adolescents experience conflict with their parents because adolescents:

MC/Mod
Pg:562
kind:c
Ans:(a)

   a) experience competing needs with respect to their parents
   b) are insecurely attached
   c) do not yet have a stable identity
   d) are in a stage of despair

16.21: Research in which beepers were used to signal adolescents and adults at various times to assess their emotional states shows that compared to adults, young people between the ages of 13 and 18:

MC/Mod
Pg:562
kind:f
Ans:(a)

   a) have more intense moods than adults
   b) show similar emotional experiences to adults
   c) have less intense moods than adults
   d) have more stable moods than adults

16.22: Based on Erikson's ideas, Marcia categorized different styles of coping with identity conflicts. One of these categories is identity diffusion. A teen with identity diffusion:

MC/Diff
Pg:563
kind:c
Ans:(a)

   a) is not actively seeking new adult roles
   b) never questioned his childhood identity
   c) is actively searching for new adult roles
   d) is in the middle of an identity crisis

16.23: At age 5, Joseph decided to become a priest. By age 20 he had never considered any other options or questioned his earlier decision. This is a style of coping with identity conflict called:

MC/Diff
Pg:563
kind:a
Ans:(b)

   a) identity diffusion
   b) identity foreclosure
   c) identity moratorium
   d) identity achievement

16.24: Which of the following describes the relationship between socioeconomic status and identity achievement?

MC/Diff
Pg:564
kind:c
Ans:(b)

    a) there is no association
    b) limited job opportunities can hinder identity achievement
    c) college students today have alienated identity achievement
    d) poorer adolescents appear not to experience identity crisis

16.25: In the 1960s, many college students were considered to have an identity status called alienated identity achievement. This meant that they:

MC/Mod
Pg:564
kind:c
Ans:(d)

    a) did not assume an adult role
    b) remained in a period of moratorium
    c) experienced identity diffusion
    d) had an adult identity which conflicted with society's values

16.26: Barbara's parents continue to provide support and guidance throughout her teenage years, but also allow her to make many of her own decisions. With this type of balanced parenting, Barbara is likely to show:

MC/Easy
Pg:564
kind:a
Ans:(b)

    a) identity diffusion
    b) identity achievement
    c) identity foreclosure
    d) alienated identity achievement

16.27: Erikson's views on adult psychosocial development have been criticized for:

MC/Mod
Pg:564
kind:c
Ans:(d)

    a) ignoring old age
    b) focusing on conflicts rather than pleasant aspects of growth
    c) ignoring intrapsychic processes
    d) ignoring the importance of relationships for women's identity

16.28: One family transition that can be disturbing to
adults is the transition to the empty nest. This
is when:

    a) a married couple realizes they can't have
       children
    b) grandparents die and parents become the eldest
       family members
    c) adult children leave the home
    d) a divorce occurs

MC/Easy
Pg:565
kind:c
Ans:(c)

16.29: Which type of child problem has been shown to be
associated with parent conflict?

    a) schizophrenia   b) conduct problems
    c) agoraphobia   d) moratorium

MC/Mod
Pg:566
kind:c
Ans:(b)

16.30: Which of the following describes the association
between marital satisfaction and having children?

    a) marital satisfaction declines after birth of
       first child
    b) marital satisfaction increases after birth of
       first child
    c) marital satisfaction declines when adult
       children leave home
    d) marital satisfaction is highest during
       children's school years

MC/Mod
Pg:566
kind:f
Ans:(a)

16.31: Which of the following characterizes the
association between ongoing marital conflict and
other family problems?

    a) unrelated to women's risk for depression
    b) related to increased risk for agoraphobia in
       women
    c) related to fewer behavior problems in children
    d) related to more father involvement in family
       life

MC/Mod
Pg:566
kind:c
Ans:(b)

16.32: Which of the following typifies the communication
styles of distressed couples?

    a) similar to nondistressed couples
    b) more positive reciprocity
    c) more negative reciprocity
    d) less clear boundaries than in nondistressed
       couples

MC/Mod
Pg:566
kind:c
Ans:(c)

16.33: Lorna Benjamin has classified relationships based on dimensions of affiliation and interdependence, to describe friendly and hostile enmeshment and differentiation. This conceptualization is based on whose theory of personality?

MC/Mod
Pg:567
kind:c
Ans:(c)

   a) Bowlby
   c) Sullivan
   b) Freud
   d) Erikson

16.34: A scapegoating pattern of family relationships is one where one family member:

MC/Mod
Pg:567
kind:c
Ans:(b)

   a) takes on all the responsibility for solving the family's problems
   b) is blamed for all the family problems
   c) bullies another family member out of jealousy
   d) complains of problems that are denied by other family members

16.35: Which is true about marriage and divorce in the U.S. today?

MC/Mod
Pg:568
kind:f
Ans:(d)

   a) Blacks are more likely to remarry than Whites after divorce
   b) about 50% of adults get married at some point in their life
   c) about 75% of marriages end in divorce
   d) most divorces happen early in the marriage

16.36: Which of the following is an example of how environments are partially heritable?

MC/Diff
Pg:568
kind:a
Ans:(d)

   a) a child is raised in her parents' home
   b) communities are segregated by socioeconomic status
   c) one's genetic background is related to one's cultural background
   d) a shy person chooses to work in a library

16.37: Behavior geneticists study the concordance rates of
monozygotic (MZ) and dizygotic (DZ) twins to
evaluate the environmental and genetic influences
on behavior. Which of the following provides
evidence for an environmental impact on behavior?

      MC/Diff
      Pg:569
      kind:f
      Ans:(a)

    a) MZ concordance rates less than 100%
    b) DZ concordance rates less than 100%
    c) MZ concordance rates greater than DZ
       concordance rates
    d) DZ concordance rates greater than MZ
       concordance rates

16.38: One limitation in the use of a heritability ratio
is that:

      MC/Diff
      Pg:569
      kind:c
      Ans:(b)

    a) it reflects only theoretically diverse
       environments
    b) it cannot be generalized to the whole
       population
    c) it can only be used to describe biological
       characteristics
    d) its calculation ignores environmental variance
       in a sample

16.39: Gottman, a researcher on marital interaction, has
described one pattern of problematic communication
called stonewalling. This involves one partner:

      MC/Easy
      Pg:570
      kind:f
      Ans:(d)

    a) denying responsibility
    b) being insulting
    c) attacking the other's personality rather than
       actions
    d) showing isolation and withdrawal

16.40: Based on observations of marital interactions,
Gottman classified four problematic communication
styles. One of these is contempt. Contempt is
characterized by:

      MC/Easy
      Pg:570
      kind:c
      Ans:(d)

    a) disinterest
    b) denying responsibility
    c) isolation and withdrawal
    d) angry insults

16.41: Which process is thought to mediate the genetic influences on divorce?

MC/Mod
Pg:571
kind:c
Ans:(c)

    a) divorced couples produce fewer offspring
    b) people who are twins rarely divorce
    c) genes influence personality traits associated with divorce
    d) unmarried couples reproduce at lower rates than married couples

16.42: One way genes are thought to affect the probability of divorce is through their expression in personality. One personality type that has a higher than average probability of divorce is:

MC/Mod
Pg:571
kind:c
Ans:(d)

    a) inhibited personality
    b) dependent personality
    c) borderline personality
    d) antisocial personality

16.43: Which of the following is true about the genetics of divorce?

MC/Mod
Pg:571
kind:f
Ans:(c)

    a) events such as marriage and divorce are unrelated to genetics
    b) divorce is more influenced by genes now than in the past
    c) concordance rates for divorce are higher in MZ than DZ twins
    d) it is impossible to estimate genetic contributions to divorce

16.44: Besides genetic contributions, one reason that concordance rates for divorce are higher among monozygotic (MZ) than dizygotic (DZ) twins may be:

MC/Mod
Pg:572
kind:c
Ans:(a)

    a) greater social disinhibition in MZ twins
    b) greater social disinhibition in DZ twins
    c) a higher divorce rate among parents of MZ twins
    d) a higher divorce rate among parents of DZ twins

16.45: Research on the Premarital Relationship Enhancement   MC/Mod
Program (PREP), where couples meet in small groups   Pg:572
to discuss marital relations and to learn   kind:c
communication skills, shows: Ans:(b)

a) little effect on marital satisfaction
b) higher marital satisfaction than control
   couples
c) more satisfaction, but also more conflict than
   controls
d) less marital satisfaction than controls 3 years
   later

16.46: Which of the following is true about formal   MC/Easy
prevention programs for life cycle transitions?   Pg:573
                                                          kind:f
a) they typically focus only on marriage   Ans:(d)
b) they must be well researched to be court
   mandated
c) they rarely involve support groups
d) they lack systematic research

16.47: Typically, a marital therapist's work involves   MC/Mod
helping spouses: Pg:573
                                                          kind:c
a) identify and voice disagreements   Ans:(a)
b) avoid disagreements and focus on the positive
c) address one partner's problem behavior
d) save their marriage and avoid divorce

16.48: Which of the following describes the effectiveness   MC/Mod
of behavioral marital therapy that addresses   Pg:574
communication styles and problem solving?   kind:f
                                                          Ans:(a)
a) as effective as other treatment approaches
b) significant short term improvement in nearly
   100% of couples
c) very little relapse
d) less effective than individual therapy

16.49: Behavioral marital therapy focuses on: MC/Easy
                                                          Pg:574
a) improving the couple's communication style   kind:c
b) changing one partner's psychopathology   Ans:(a)
c) changing how parents act toward their troubled
   child
d) talking about the marriage in individual
   therapy

322

16.50: An improved marriage helps to alleviate individual
disorders. Although this is true for many
disorders, it appears most true for:

a) anxiety
c) depression
b) alcoholism
d) schizophrenia

MC/Mod
Pg:574
kind:f
Ans:(c)

16.51: The cessation of menstruation is called:

a) moratorium
c) menopause
b) menarche
d) midlife crisis

MC/Easy
Pg:574
kind:f
Ans:(c)

16.52: Hormone replacement therapy during menopause is
effective for reducing:

a) depression
b) risk of cancer
c) infertility
d) emotional volatility

MC/Mod
Pg:575
kind:f
Ans:(d)

16.53: Some women experience depression during menopause.
Depression during menopause is associated with:

a) decreased estrogen
b) increased estrogen
c) changes in roles and identity
d) calcium depletion

MC/Mod
Pg:575
kind:f
Ans:(c)

16.54: Bereavement is:

a) a process of coping with any separation or loss
b) a period of adjustment to old age
c) a specific form of grief about death
d) a form of clinical depression

MC/Mod
Pg:576
kind:c
Ans:(c)

16.55: Mrs. Pallagio's husband dies at age 70. For the
next year, she finds herself thinking about him
constantly. Every night she talks out loud to his
photo. A clinical psychologist would describe
these behaviors as:

a) a normal part of grieving
b) a sign of abnormal obsessionality
c) a sign of delusional thinking
d) evidence of an abnormal lack of anger

MC/Mod
Pg:576
kind:a
Ans:(a)

16.56: Elisabeth Kubler-Ross is known for her ideas on:

    a) children's grief after separation from a caregiver
    b) terminally ill patients' emotions about dying
    c) adolescent identity crisis
    d) the midlife crisis

MC/Easy
Pg:576
kind:f
Ans:(b)

16.57: Bowlby based his model of bereavement on attachment theory and observations of children who had lost their parent. Kubler-Ross based her model on observations of the terminally ill. One stage that Kubler-Ross included that is not part of Bowlby's model is:

    a) bargaining
    b) denial
    c) depression
    d) reorganization and acceptance

MC/Mod
Pg:577
kind:c
Ans:(a)

16.58: An element that is important in both Bowlby's and Kubler-Ross' models of bereavement is:

    a) anger   b) bargaining
    c) moratorium   d) identity crisis

MC/Mod
Pg:577
kind:c
Ans:(a)

16.59: Evidence on bereavement shows that mourners:

    a) vacillate between different emotions and "stages"
    b) go through a fixed sequence of stages of grief
    c) show sadness but little anger
    d) show better adjustment if bereavement is intense

MC/Mod
Pg:577
kind:c
Ans:(a)

16.60: A grandfather who reminisces out loud about how his Irish parents celebrated holidays, and who tells stories from his childhood about lessons he learned, is engaging in a type of reminiscence called:

    a) escapist   b) integrative
    c) instrumental   d) transitive

MC/Mod
Pg:578
kind:a
Ans:(d)

16.61: Research on different styles of reminiscence in   MC/Mod
       older adults has found adjustment to be least   Pg:578
       successful when reminiscence is: kind:f
                                                           Ans:(d)
       a) integrative   b) instrumental
       c) transitive   d) obsessive

16.62: A disorder that is more prominent among the elderly MC/Easy
       is: Pg:578
                                                           kind:f
       a) cognitive disorder   b) depression   Ans:(a)
       c) anxiety   d) schizophrenia

16.63: Which of the following is true about the symptoms   MC/Diff
       of depression in the elderly?   Pg:578
                                                           kind:f
       a) the depression is less severe than that found   Ans:(b)
          in younger people
       b) the suicide rate is highest among the elderly
       c) depression is more common among the elderly
       d) depression in the elderly is mostly due to
          bereavement

16.64: Ageism refers to: MC/Easy
                                                           Pg:578
       a) the incorporation of age norms in research   kind:f
       b) changes as one grows older   Ans:(d)
       c) the study of aging and the elderly
       d) prejudice against the elderly

16.65: Research on the elderly shows older people's   MC/Mod
       personality to be: Pg:578
                                                           kind:c
       a) less inwardly focused   Ans:(d)
       b) more irritable and complaining
       c) greatly affected by depression and anxiety
       d) similar to the personality shown in middle age

16.66: The multidisciplinary study of aging is known as: MC/Easy
                                                           Pg:578
       a) ageism   b) moratorium studies   kind:f
       c) life cycle studies   d) gerontology   Ans:(d)

325

16.67: Gerontologists classify the people as young-old, old-old, and oldest-old. The oldest-old are those over age:

a) 55
b) 65
c) 75
d) 85

MC/Easy
Pg:579
kind:f
Ans:(d)

16.68: In gerontology, the classification of young-old is defined by:

a) age over 65
b) age in the 60s and 70s, in good health
c) young adults with health problems and stubborn personalities
d) young adults in nursing homes

MC/Mod
Pg:579
kind:c
Ans:(b)

16.69: About what percentage of the oldest-old (those over age 85) live in nursing homes?

a) 10%
b) 22%
c) 50%
d) 72%

MC/Mod
Pg:579
kind:f
Ans:(b)

16.70: Most elderly people fall in which category?

a) young
b) young-old
c) old-old
d) oldest-old

MC/Mod
Pg:579
kind:f
Ans:(b)

16.71: The biggest trend in the average age of the U.S. population in the next 40 years is due to:

a) divorce and remarriage resulting in more children and a younger population
b) immigration of young families resulting in a younger population
c) baby boom generation reaching old age
d) medical advances increasing the number of older and frail adults

MC/Mod
Pg:579
kind:c
Ans:(c)

16.72: The proportion of the U.S. population aged 65 and older should peak around the year:

a) 2000
b) 2015
c) 2030
d) 2045

MC/Mod
Pg:579
kind:f
Ans:(c)

16.73: Which of the following typifies the living conditions of the elderly?

    a) the majority of elderly men live alone
    b) the majority of elderly women live alone
    c) most elderly live in nursing homes
    d) elderly widows have higher than average economic status

MC/Mod
Pg:579
kind:f
Ans:(b)

16.74: Which is a social factor thought to moderate the ill effects of bereavement?

    a) avoidance of remarriage
    b) moving into a nursing home
    c) religious affiliation and involvement
    d) family members encouraging self-sufficiency

MC/Mod
Pg:580
kind:c
Ans:(c)

16.75: Behavioral gerontology is a new subdiscipline devoted to treating behavior problems among:

    a) children   b) adolescent
    c) adults   d) the elderly

MC/Easy
Pg:581
kind:f
Ans:(d)

True-False Questions

16.76: Life cycle transitions are not mental disorders.

TF/Easy
Pg:556
kind:f
Ans:True

16.77: Erikson believed that psychosocial development reached stagnation by young adulthood.

TF/Easy
Pg:558
kind:f
Ans:False

16.78: Periods of life cycle transition are usually characterized by low interpersonal conflict.

TF/Easy
Pg:558
kind:f
Ans:False

16.79: According to Erikson, forming an intimate relationship is not an important task of early adulthood.

TF/Mod
Pg:559
kind:f
Ans:False

16.80: According to Erikson, normal adolescence is a period of confusion and uncertainty.

TF/Easy
Pg:561
kind:f
Ans:True

16.81: In normal development, young adults want independence from their parents and do not want their parents' support.

TF/Easy
Pg:562
kind:f
Ans:False

16.82: Adolescents in the middle of an identity crisis are in a period of moratorium.

TF/Mod
Pg:562
kind:c
Ans:True

16.83: Identity diffusion can result from having limited occupational opportunities.

TF/Diff
Pg:564
kind:c
Ans:True

16.84: Women in traditional sex roles typically form an identity and then, based on this identity, enter into relationships with others.

TF/Mod
Pg:565
kind:c
Ans:False

16.85: Models of the family life cycle are typically conceptualized in terms of changes in household composition or relationships.

TF/Easy
Pg:565
kind:c
Ans:True

16.86: Ongoing marital conflict is associated with increased risk for depression and agoraphobia in women.

TF/Easy
Pg:566
kind:f
Ans:True

16.87: For women, there is a higher risk of depression associated with ongoing family conflict than with divorce.

TF/Easy
Pg:566
kind:f
Ans:True

16.88: Only about 25% of all of today's marriages will end in divorce.

TF/Easy
Pg:568
kind:f
Ans:False

16.89: Distressed and nondistressed couples show similar communication patterns.

TF/Easy
Pg:568
kind:f
Ans:False

16.90: Heritability is the proportion of variance in a trait that is attributable to genetic factors.

TF/Easy
Pg:569
kind:f
Ans:True

16.91: Divorce is thought to be partly genetic, because some personality characteristics are influenced by genetics and also predispose to divorce.

TF/Mod
Pg:571
kind:c
Ans:True

16.92: The most common programs for promoting marital success are provided by religious groups.

TF/Easy
Pg:572
kind:f
Ans:True

16.93: Marital therapists help couples avoid disagreements and focus on positive aspects of the relationship.

TF/Mod
Pg:573
kind:f
Ans:False

16.94: Individual therapy for each spouse is more effective than marital therapy in most cases.

TF/Mod
Pg:574
kind:f
Ans:False

16.95: Menopause is characterized by the cessation of menstruation.

TF/Easy
Pg:574
kind:f
Ans:True

16.96: It is normal for intense grief over the death of a loved one to continue for a year or two.

TF/Easy
Pg:576
kind:f
Ans:True

16.97: Anger is a natural and normal part of grief.

TF/Easy
Pg:577
kind:c
Ans:True

16.98: The prevalence of mental disorders is higher among   TF/Mod
       the elderly.   Pg:578
                                                               kind:f
                                                               Ans:False

16.99: The majority of older adults are classified as   TF/Mod
       "young-old" and show physical health and vigor.   Pg:579
                                                               kind:f
                                                               Ans:True

16.100: Bereavement and living alone are more strongly   TF/Mod
        related to depression among women than among men.   Pg:580
                                                               kind:f
                                                               Ans:False

16.101: Electroconvulsive therapy (ECT) may be more   TF/Mod
        effective for treating severe depression in the   Pg:581
        elderly than in younger adults.   kind:f
                                                               Ans:True

Essay Questions

16.102: Why are life cycle transitions of interest to clinical
        psychologists?

Answer: Many people seek help during challenging times, even if their
        disturbance does not constitute a mental disorder. However, life
        stressors can also contribute to the etiology of a mental
        disorder, especially if the person shows inadequate coping with
        the stress. For example, Freud believed that depression is caused
        by inadequate resolution of grief.

        ES   Easy   Page: 556   kind: c

16.103: Theories on stages of adult psychosocial development are useful, but must be considered with caution. Explain why.

Answer: Each theory was developed in cultural, historical, and personal contexts that influence the definition of what is normal. Although these theories usually describe adult development as occurring in a sequence of stages, research shows that the order of

transitions is not predictable. Once the problems of one stage are resolved, they may again become problems later. Finally, there is evidence that men and women might follow different developmental paths, but these differences typically are not addressed by stage theories of adult development.

ES   Moderate   Page: 560   kind: c

16.104: What is the crosscultural evidence on adolescent identity crisis?

Answer: An identity crisis during adolescence may be a phenomenon limited to modern industrialized societies. Affluence, education, and alternative make options possible. In less developed countries, one's role is often decided by one's parents or economic pressures and lack of options.

ES   Moderate   Page: 564   kind: c

16.105: Describe the type of emotional reciprocity found in families with happy relationships compared to those found in families with troubled relationships.

Answer: Happy families reciprocate pleasantness and ignore negativity. Troubled families ignore pleasantness or see it as manipulative, and reciprocate negativity.

ES   Moderate   Page: 566   kind: c

16.106: Discuss the various explanations for research results showing that happily married individuals show lower rates of psychopathology than average.

Answer: Individual psychopathology may induce distress in a marriage. Alternatively, distressed marriages may produce individual psychopathology. A satisfying marriage may be a factor that protects individuals from psychopathology. Finally, psychopathological individuals are more likely to be unmarried or divorced.

ES   Moderate   Page: 571   kind: c

16.107: Explain how attachment theory explains why someone might feel angry in the middle of intense sadness over a loss.

Answer: When alive, the attachment figure was signalled to reunion when the child expressed protest and the attachment figure was close. Anger and protect after the attachment figure's death is similarly evoked.

ES Moderate Page: 577 kind: c

16.108: What evidence from studies on divorce and bereavement suggests that being married may be more important for men's happiness than for women's happiness?

Answer: Divorce increases the probability of depression in men, whereas marital dissatisfaction (not divorce) increases depression in women. Losing a spouse through death results in more depression for men than women.

ES Moderate Page: 580 kind: c

Chapter 17
Mental Health and the Law

Multiple Choice Questions

17.1: Criminal law assumes that human behavior is the product of free will. This means that:

    a) people make choices and are responsible for them
    b) behavior is determined by social, biological, and psychological forces
    c) human behavior is animalistic and needs regulation
    d) laws are needed because most people don't know right from wrong

MC/Easy
Pg:588
kind:c
Ans:(a)

17.2: Criminal responsibility rests on the concept of:

    a) determinism
    b) free will
    c) humanism
    d) moral treatment

MC/Easy
Pg:588
kind:c
Ans:(b)

17.3: In contrast to the legal system's philosophy of human behavior, most mental health professionals assume that human behavior is:

    a) a product of personal choice and free will
    b) ultimately the individual's responsibility
    c) determined by biological, social, and psychological forces
    d) basically good, and without need of laws

MC/Mod
Pg:588
kind:c
Ans:(c)

17.4: In order to conduct scientific research, it is essential for psychologists to make an assumption of:

    a) free will
    b) determinism
    c) reasonable doubt
    d) personal responsibility

MC/Mod
Pg:588
kind:c
Ans:(b)

17.5: Under U.S. law, the legally insane individual is
assumed:

    a) not to be entitled to constitutional
       protections
    b) not to be acting out of free will
    c) to be criminally responsible
    d) to be suffering from schizophrenia

MC/Mod
Pg:588
kind:c
Ans:(b)

17.6: According to psychiatrist Thomas Szasz, people are
labeled "mentally ill" because:

    a) they have a psychiatric illness
    b) they don't have free will
    c) they don't fit into society
    d) they are not responsible for their actions

MC/Mod
Pg:589
kind:c
Ans:(c)

17.7: Thomas Szasz has argued that the insanity defense
should be abolished because:

    a) the mentally ill should not be tried
    b) the insane do not have free will
    c) the mentally ill do not understand the legal
       system
    d) all people are responsible for their actions

MC/Mod
Pg:589
kind:c
Ans:(d)

17.8: Thomas Szasz believes that the label of mental
illness is applied to people who are not diseased
but who are instead socially deviant. In its
extreme, this labeling is associated with broad
social abuses such as:

    a) the abolishment of the insanity defense
    b) the ready availability of antipsychotic
       medications
    c) the mentally ill being denied insurance
       coverage
    d) the confinement of political dissidents in
       hospitals

MC/Mod
Pg:589
kind:c
Ans:(d)

17.9: A persistent problem with the insanity defense and the verdict of "not guilty by reason of insanity" (NGRI) is:

MC/Mod
Pg:590
kind:c
Ans:(c)

a) there is no burden of proof to demonstrate sanity
b) if the person is found NGRI, he or she still goes to prison
c) expert testimony about sanity is often contradictory
d) if the person if found NGRI, he or she receives no treatment

17.10: Before the 1800s, acquittals due to the "insanity" of the defendant were based on the idea that the defendant:

MC/Mod
Pg:590
kind:c
Ans:(a)

a) did not know right from wrong
b) experienced an irresistible impulse
c) showed behavior that was the product of mental illness
d) did not have the burden of proof

17.11: M'Naghten was a British subject who claimed that the "voice of God" told him to kill the Prime Minister in the 1840s. He was acquitted because of insanity. The reasons for this acquittal came to be known as the M'Naghten test, which is whether or not the defendant:

MC/Mod
Pg:590
kind:c
Ans:(b)

a) experiences an irresistible impulse
b) knows right from wrong
c) shows behavior that is the product of mental illness
d) has the burden of proving insanity

17.12: In the late 19th century, defendants could be found not guilty be reason of insanity if they were unable to control their impulses because of mental disease. The rationale for the irresistible impulse test was that:

MC/Diff
Pg:590
kind:c
Ans:(d)

a) everyone knows right from wrong
b) the M'Naghten test was too broad
c) some diagnoses are based on evidence of criminal behavior
d) conviction can not deter uncontrollable behavior

17.13: The effect of the product test in determining verdicts of "not guilty by reason of insanity" (NGRI) was to:

    a) reduce the number of NGRI verdicts
    b) acknowledge the ineffectiveness of deterrence in some cases
    c) establish if the person knows right from wrong
    d) allow mental health professionals wide discretion in determining insanity

MC/Mod
Pg:590
kind:c
Ans:(d)

17.14: The most ENDURING standard for declaring a person not guilty by reason of insanity (NGRI) has been:

    a) the M'Naghten rule
    b) the irresistible impulse test
    c) the product test
    d) diagnosis of antisocial personality disorder

MC/Mod
Pg:591
kind:c
Ans:(a)

17.15: A new verdict, in place in about a quarter of the states, is "Guilty but Mentally Ill." Persons who receive this verdict:

    a) are not convicted
    b) must be legally insane at the time of the offense
    c) fail the M'Naghten test
    d) are convicted but also are ordered to receive treatment

MC/Mod
Pg:591
kind:c
Ans:(d)

17.16: Among the categories of mental disease that are generally EXCLUDED from consideration as part of an insanity defense is:

    a) schizophrenia   b) affective disorders
    c) mental retardation   d) substance abuse

MC/Mod
Pg:592
kind:f
Ans:(d)

17.17: One reason why many mental health professionals do not think that they should testify as to whether or not a defendant is insane is that:

    a) insanity is a legal, not psychological, concept
    b) the defendant might not go to prison
    c) their answer might not be in the client's best interest
    d) they are not given enough diagnostic information to make a decision

MC/Mod
Pg:592
kind:c
Ans:(a)

17.18: Defendants found not guilty by reason of insanity   MC/Mod
(NGRI) are sent to a hospital rather than a jail.   Pg:593
On average, the amount of time they spend in the   kind:f
hospital is: Ans:(b)

   a) shorter than the time they would have spent in
      jail
   b) about the same as the amount of time they would
      have spent in jail
   c) longer than the amount of time they would have
      spent in jail
   d) so long as to be virtually a lifetime sentence

17.19: If a person is found incompetent to stand trial,   MC/Mod
what happens?   Pg:593
    kind:c
   a) the charges are dismissed   Ans:(d)
   b) the person is found not guilty by reason of
      incompetence
   c) the person is found not guilty by reason of
      insanity
   d) proceedings are postponed until the person is
      competent

17.20: Competence refers to the defendant's ability to   MC/Diff
understand the proceedings taking place and to: Pg:593
    kind:c
   a) participate in their own defense   Ans:(a)
   b) pay for a lawyer
   c) remember what happened at the time of the crime
   d) be nonpsychotic

17.21: In order to be found competent to stand trial, a   MC/Easy
defendant must: Pg:593
    kind:f
   a) understand the charges   Ans:(a)
   b) know right from wrong
   c) be nonpsychotic
   d) be willing to meet with a lawyer

17.22: A person found to be incompetent to stand trial is: MC/Mod
    Pg:593
   a) sent home and the proceedings are dropped   kind:f
   b) sent to jail until found to be competent   Ans:(c)
   c) sent to the hospital until found to be
      competent
   d) institutionalized for an amount of time
      comparable to a likely sentence

17.23: Most people who are determined to be incompetent are determined to be incompetent at what time point?

    a) at the time of the arrest
    b) at the time of sentencing
    c) when it is time to stand trial
    d) when they are about to be executed

MC/Easy
Pg:594
kind:f
Ans:(c)

17.24: Competence refers to the defendant's mental state during what time period?

    a) at any point in the legal process
    b) only at the time of the offense
    c) only at the time of arrest
    d) only at the time of the trial

MC/Mod
Pg:594
kind:c
Ans:(a)

17.25: The defense of "Not Guilty by Reason of Insanity" (NGRI) is used in about what percentage of cases?

    a) 1%   b) 5%
    c) 10%   d) 25%

MC/Easy
Pg:595
kind:f
Ans:(a)

17.26: Dorothea Dix (1802-1887) was known for:

    a) initiating the deinstitutionalization movement
    b) discovering the first antipsychotic medications
    c) accusing the mentally ill of being witches
    d) advocating humane treatment of the mentally ill

MC/Mod
Pg:595
kind:f
Ans:(d)

17.27: The moral treatment movement was associated with:

    a) a view of the mentally ill as needing religious training
    b) deinstitutionalization
    c) humanistic institutions for the mentally ill
    d) the development of the insanity defense

MC/Mod
Pg:595
kind:c
Ans:(c)

17.28: Many of the terrible conditions of many modern mental hospitals were disclosed in the 1940s by:

    a) patients who improved on medications
    b) nurses who protested
    c) conscientious objectors working in the hospitals
    d) government officials looking for cost-efficient programs

MC/Mod
Pg:595
kind:c
Ans:(c)

17.29: The deinstitutionalization movement began around: MC/Easy
                                                                        Pg:596
   a) 1800   b) 1850   kind:f
   c) 1900   d) 1950   Ans:(d)

17.30: The procedure for admitting a patient to a   MC/Easy
       psychiatric hospital involuntarily is known as: Pg:596
                                                                        kind:f
   a) civil commitment   Ans:(a)
   b) libertarian commitment
   c) deinstitutionalization
   d) parens patriae

17.31: One justification for civil commitment to   MC/Mod
       psychiatric hospitals is the philosophy of parens   Pg:596
       patriae. This is the government's responsibility   kind:c
       to: Ans:(b)

   a) keep the mentally ill from having children
   b) protect and care for society's weaker members
   c) provide police power and protection for society
      at large
   d) reimburse family members who care for the
      mentally ill

17.32: Which of the following is true about the civil   MC/Mod
       commitment procedures in the late 1800s?   Pg:597
                                                                        kind:f
   a) a husband could commit his wife even if she was   Ans:(a)
      not mentally ill
   b) there were no psychiatric hospitals to which
      people could be committed
   c) the mentally ill were committed to jails
   d) the M'Naghten rule determined if a person could
      be legally committed

17.33: Today, the emergency commitment procedures in most   MC/Mod
       states allow an acutely disturbed individual to be: Pg:597
                                                                        kind:f
   a) confined to a mental hospital for a few days   Ans:(a)
   b) confined to a mental hospital until treatment
      is finished
   c) confined to a jail for a few days
   d) confined to a jail until the person agrees to
      be treated

17.34: Which of the following describes the civil rights of patients committed to psychiatric hospitals?

MC/Mod
Pg:597
kind:c
Ans:(a)

a) their due process rights must be protected
b) civil rights protection becomes a medical, not a legal, concern
c) committed patients lose all of their civil rights
d) committed patients must be read their Miranda rights

17.35: A person can be committed to a psychiatric hospital for various reasons. One reason that has been criticized on philosophical grounds for being paternalistic is:

MC/Mod
Pg:597
kind:c
Ans:(d)

a) dangerousness to self
b) dangerousness to others
c) incompetency
d) inability to care for self

17.36: Which of the following describes the rate of violence among patients with bipolar disorder, major depression, and schizophrenia?

MC/Mod
Pg:598
kind:f
Ans:(d)

a) the rate is much lower than in the general population
b) the rate is about the same as the general population
c) violence almost always occurs during episodes of illness
d) the rate is about 5 times higher than the general population

17.37: Clinical assessments are often used to predict whether an individual will be violent if released from the hospital. About how often do these assessments result in accurate predictions?

MC/Diff
Pg:598
kind:f
Ans:(a)

a) they are right at above-chance levels
b) they are right about 2 out of 3 times
c) they are wrong 99% of the time
d) they are right 99% of the time

17.38: According to the results of Lidz, Mulvey, and
Gardner's (1993) study of clinical predictions of
violence, clinicians:

    a) are more accurate at predicting women's
       violence than men's
    b) can predict men's violence at
       better-than-chance levels
    c) are not able to predict violence at
       better-than-chance levels
    d) can predict violence only if there is
       information on past violence

MC/Mod
Pg:599
kind:c
Ans:(b)

17.39: To improve past research, Lidz, Mulvey, and Gardner
(1993) placed a greater emphasis on getting
information about patients' violent behavior from:

    a) court records
    b) hospital records
    c) police reports
    d) interviews with patients and family members

MC/Mod
Pg:599
kind:c
Ans:(d)

17.40: The accuracy of predictions about future events
depends in part on the base rate of the event. The
base rate is:

    a) the number of guesses made about the event
    b) how frequently the event occurs
    c) the amount of information available to make a
       prediction
    d) the accuracy of predictions about the event in
       the past

MC/Mod
Pg:600
kind:c
Ans:(b)

17.41: The percentage of patients who commit acts of
violence is highest among patients with which type
of disorder?

    a) major depression   b) bipolar disorder
    c) schizophrenia   d) substance abuse

MC/Mod
Pg:600
kind:f
Ans:(d)

17.42: Inaccurate predictions of violence and suicide risk
are especially likely to show:

    a) high true positive rates
    b) high true negative rates
    c) high false negative rates
    d) high false positive rates

MC/Mod
Pg:600
kind:f
Ans:(d)

17.43: Which is true about the commitment of children to psychiatric hospitals?

    a) children are entitled to a hearing before being committed
    b) parents cannot commit a child without a court hearing
    c) parents can commit a child against the child's wishes
    d) children do not need parental permission to check themselves out of the hospital

MC/Mod
Pg:601
kind:f
Ans:(c)

17.44: Based on her study of adolescents in psychiatric hospitals, Weithorn (1988) concluded that the adolescent inpatient population:

    a) shows more serious psychopathology than in the past
    b) included more status offenders who used to go through the courts
    c) has decreased in the 1980s
    d) has more due process protection than before

MC/Diff
Pg:601
kind:c
Ans:(c)

17.45: The case of Wyatt v. Stickney (1972), a legal battle between a hospitalized psychiatric patient and the Alabama Mental Health Commissioner, established for patients the basic right of:

    a) treatment in the least restrictive environment
    b) refusing treatment
    c) treatment while hospitalized
    d) review of commitment every 6 months

MC/Diff
Pg:601
kind:f
Ans:(c)

17.46: When Supreme Court Justice Blackmun heard that the prediction of violence is wrong 2 out of 3 times, he concluded that predicting violence using a coin flip would be more accurate. He was wrong because:

    a) the coin flip is random, not based on clinical judgment
    b) the base rate of violence is much lower than 50%
    c) the specificity of a coin flip is above 50%
    d) the sensitivity of a coin flip is above 50%

MC/Diff
Pg:602
kind:c
Ans:(b)

17.47: In O'Connor v. Donaldson (1975), a patient who had been confined in a hospital for 15 years argued that he was being deprived of his constitutional right to liberty. The court decided that patients cannot be confined against their will if they:

   a) are taking medications as prescribed
   b) have a home to go to
   c) are not dangerous to themselves or others
   d) have an outpatient therapist

17.48: The legal case of Lake v. Cameron concerned an elderly women who had a cognitive disorder that caused her to wander from her home. She was confined to a hospital because of her cognitive disorder. In this legal decision, the court decided that she:

   a) could not be confined without treatment
   b) could not be confined if not dangerous
   c) must be treated in the least restrictive environment
   d) had the right to refuse treatment

17.49: The most important issue about the least restrictive environment alternative is:

   a) treatment in a less restrictive environment is usually less effective
   b) less restrictive environments are often not available
   c) insurance companies won't pay the expenses for alternative treatments
   d) treatment in these settings is usually prohibitively expensive

17.50: A patient can refuse treatment if procedures of
informed consent are followed. When the patient
wants to refuse treatment but is not competent to
give consent, a common practice is to assign an
independent guardian who provides a substituted
judgment. A substituted judgment is:

MC/Mod
Pg:605
kind:f
Ans:(a)

   a) an opinion as to what the patient would have
      decided if competent
   b) a decision about what's best for the patient
   c) a decision to postpone a hearing until the
      patient is competent
   d) a proposal for a less restrictive treatment as
      a compromise

17.51: The philosophy of deinstitutionalization is that
the mentally ill and mentally retarded:

MC/Mod
Pg:605
kind:c
Ans:(a)

   a) can be better served in the community rather
      than the hospital
   b) need to be hospitalized under more humane
      conditions
   c) should be hospitalized if they are homeless
   d) should be placed in private, not public,
      hospitals

17.52: In 1963, the Community Mental Health Center act was
passed in an effort to provide:

MC/Mod
Pg:605
kind:c
Ans:(d)

   a) information and legal advice about mental
      health issues
   b) programs to prevent mental illness
   c) better training for clinical psychologists
   d) an alternative to institutionalized psychiatric
      care

17.53: Community Mental Health Centers first came into
existence in the:

MC/Easy
Pg:605
kind:f
Ans:(c)

   a) 1920s   b) 1940s
   c) 1960s   d) 1980s

344

17.54: Community Mental Health Centers have not met the
       needs created by deinstitutionalization, mainly
       because:

    a) they only treat schizophrenics, not less
       disturbed patients
    b) they don't target their treatments for the
       seriously mentally ill
    c) they don't adhere to the moral treatment
       movement
    d) they cannot dispense antipsychotic medications

MC/Mod
Pg:606
kind:c
Ans:(b)

17.55: Which is true about courts for family law, such as
       juvenile courts and domestic relations courts?

    a) they were established to counteract the parens
       patriae role of government
    b) they are based on the state's police powers
    c) they provide a greater role for mental health
       professionals
    d) they were not established until the 1970s

MC/Mod
Pg:608
kind:f
Ans:(c)

17.56: Physical custody refers to:

    a) which parent makes medical and educational
       decisions about a child
    b) winning material possessions in a divorce
       settlement
    c) which parent the child lives with
    d) foster care placement of abused children

MC/Easy
Pg:608
kind:c
Ans:(c)

17.57: Research on the effects of divorce on children
       consistently shows that among children whose
       parents have divorced:

    a) there is a much higher level of psychological
       problems
    b) many psychological problems begin long before
       the divorce occurs
    c) psychological problems always start during and
       after the divorce
    d) there is no evidence of higher rates of
       psychological problems

MC/Mod
Pg:609
kind:f
Ans:(b)

17.58: Which is true about how custody decisions are made?

    a) most are settled in court by a judge
    b) they cannot be made legally through mediation
    c) they must involve a psychiatric evaluation of the parents
    d) most are made outside of the court with the aid of an attorney

MC/Mod
Pg:610
kind:f
Ans:(d)

17.59: The "child's best interest" standard for determining custody refers to:

    a) the child's expressed wishes
    b) the parents' standard of living and financial resources
    c) the idea that all children should be placed with their mother
    d) the vague notion of an optimal childrearing environment

MC/Mod
Pg:610
kind:c
Ans:(d)

17.60: Mediation to settle custody disputes is characterized by:

    a) an adversarial approach to dispute resolution
    b) a cooperative approach to dispute resolution
    c) an objective third party making a custody decision
    d) attempts to convince the parents not to divorce

MC/Mod
Pg:610
kind:c
Ans:(b)

17.61: Which of the following is true about mediation to settle child custody disputes?

    a) it increases the number of custody hearings in court
    b) parents like it less than litigation
    c) it helps parents reach a settlement more quickly
    d) it does not result in a legal agreement

MC/Mod
Pg:610
kind:f
Ans:(c)

17.62: Which is true about the rates of child abuse in the last 2 decades?

    a) the number of official reports has increased steadily
    b) the number of official reports has decreased steadily
    c) child abuse rates peaked in the 1980s
    d) actual cases of child abuse are declining

MC/Mod
Pg:611
kind:f
Ans:(a)

17.63: The first child protection efforts in the U.S.
began with the founding of the New York Society for
the Prevention of Cruelty to Children, around:

MC/Mod
Pg:611
kind:f
Ans:(c)

a) 1790
c) 1875

b) 1820
d) 1950

17.64: One of the most important consequences of Kempe's
1962 article on the battered child syndrome was:

MC/Mod
Pg:611
kind:c
Ans:(a)

a) the establishment of reporting laws
b) the delineation of 4 types of abuse
c) the differentiation of attention deficit from
neglect
d) the differentiation of physical abuse from crib
death

17.65: One reason for the great increase in the number of
reported child abuse cases in the last 2 decades is
the increasing number of:

MC/Mod
Pg:611
kind:f
Ans:(b)

a) professionals who are mandated to report
b) unsubstantiated reports
c) children reporting their own abuse
d) videocameras documenting abuse in stores and
banks

17.66: Which is true about malpractice in the mental
health professions?

MC/Mod
Pg:612
kind:f
Ans:(a)

a) a person can lose his or her license if found
guilty of malpractice
b) a person cannot be sued for malpractice if his
or her license is valid
c) sex with a client is not grounds for
malpractice
d) medication issues rarely result in malpractice
suits

17.67: Approximately what percentage of female murder
victims are killed by their husband or boyfriend?

MC/Mod
Pg:613
kind:f
Ans:(d)

a) 1%
c) 15%

b) 5%
d) 33%

347

17.68: When a woman kills her abusive husband, her legal
defense often rests on proving that she:

   a) suffered from the battered woman syndrome
   b) is not guilty by reason of insanity
   c) was influenced by the media
   d) was suffering from a major mental illness

MC/Mod
Pg:613
kind:c
Ans:(a)

17.69: According to the ethical codes of the American
Psychiatric Association and the American
Psychological Association, sexual relations between
a client and therapist are:

   a) not unethical if mutually consensual
   b) not grounds for malpractice
   c) considered damaging in and of themselves
   d) are discouraged but not prohibited

MC/Mod
Pg:615
kind:f
Ans:(c)

17.70: The legal case of Tarasoff v. Regents of the
University of California (1976) established that
therapists must:

   a) report suspected cases of child abuse
   b) notify police of a patient's imminent suicide
      attempt
   c) warn potential victims of a patient's intent to
      harm them
   d) refrain from sex with clients

MC/Mod
Pg:617
kind:f
Ans:(c)

17.71: In most states, the Tarasoff decision means that
therapists are required to notify a potential
victim of a patient's intent to harm:

   a) even if there is only a vague threat
   b) only if they can do so without breaking
      confidentiality
   c) even if the patient changes his mind and is no
      longer threatening
   d) only if there is a specific, identifiable
      target

MC/Mod
Pg:617
kind:f
Ans:(d)

True-False Questions

17.72: Free will is a scientific concept.

TF/Easy
Pg:588
kind:f
Ans:False

17.73: Thomas Szasz believes that the mentally ill should be given the same dignity and social responsibilities as the mentally healthy.

TF/Mod
Pg:589
kind:f
Ans:True

17.74: The legal definition of mental disease is less restrictive than the definition used by mental health professionals.

TF/Easy
Pg:592
kind:f
Ans:False

17.75: Most defendants who use the defense of not guilty by reason of insanity are in fact found not guilty by reason of insanity.

TF/Mod
Pg:593
kind:f
Ans:False

17.76: A psychotic individual is automatically considered incompetent to stand trial.

TF/Mod
Pg:593
kind:f
Ans:False

17.77: Among people who are accused of crimes, more are institutionalized in psychiatric hospitals because of incompetence than because of insanity.

TF/Easy
Pg:594
kind:f
Ans:True

17.78: The increased use of antipsychotic medications in the 1950s meant more patients had to stay in the hospital for longer periods than before.

TF/Easy
Pg:596
kind:f
Ans:False

17.79: Libertarian views on hospitalizing people against their will focus on the state's duty to protect citizens from mentally ill people who are dangerous.

TF/Easy
Pg:596
kind:f
Ans:False

17.80: In the past, it was much easier to commit someone to a mental hospital than it is now.

TF/Easy
Pg:597
kind:f
Ans:True

17.81: The prevalence of bipolar disorder, major depression, and schizophrenia is not higher among prison inmates than it is among the general population.

TF/Mod
Pg:598
kind:f
Ans:False

17.82: Research suggests that clinicians are more accurate at predicting men's future violence than they are at predicting women's future violence.

TF/Mod
Pg:599
kind:f
Ans:True

17.83: After the court case of Wyatt v. Stickney, which established patients' right to treatment while hospitalized, many patients were released because they could not all be treated up to standard in overcrowded hospitals.

TF/Mod
Pg:603
kind:f
Ans:True

17.84: Only 1 or 2 states allow patients to refuse psychotropic medications if involuntarily committed to the hospital.

TF/Mod
Pg:605
kind:f
Ans:False

17.85: One problem with Community Mental Health Centers is that they don't offer many services for the seriously mentally ill.

TF/Mod
Pg:606
kind:c
Ans:True

17.86: About 1% of the homeless are mentally ill.

TF/Easy
Pg:606
kind:f
Ans:False

17.87: There are more mentally ill individuals living on the streets and in shelters than in public mental hospitals.

TF/Mod
Pg:606
kind:f
Ans:True

17.88: Family law cases such as divorce and adoption are handled in different courts than are civil commitment cases.

TF/Easy
Pg:607
kind:f
Ans:True

17.89: Divorce is more common among African-Americans than among European-Americans.

TF/Easy
Pg:608
kind:f
Ans:True

17.90: On average, children whose parents have divorced show only slightly more psychological problems than children of married parents.

TF/Mod
Pg:609
kind:f
Ans:True

17.91: The standard of "the child's best interests" in determining custody refers to the child's expressed wishes about which parent he or she would like to live with.

TF/Easy
Pg:610
kind:c
Ans:False

17.92: In most states, the reporting requirement with respect to child abuse is that physicians, mental health professionals, and teachers must report suspected child abuse to the authorities.

TF/Mod
Pg:611
kind:f
Ans:True

17.93: Legally, negligence is substandard professional service, but does not necessarily result in harm to clients or patients.

TF/Easy
Pg:612
kind:f
Ans:True

17.94: In some states, it is not considered rape if a husband forces his wife to have sex with him.

TF/Easy
Pg:613
kind:f
Ans:True

17.95: Psychiatrists have among the highest rates of malpractice of all medical specialties.

TF/Mod
Pg:614
kind:f
Ans:False

17.96: Mental health professionals are required to break confidentiality if necessary to report cases of suspected child abuse.

TF/Mod
Pg:616
kind:f
Ans:True

Essay Questions

17.97: What changes in the "not guilty by reason of insanity" (NGRI) defense were made as a result of the case of John Hinckley, who shot President Reagan?

Answer: After the Hinckley case, the presence of an irresistible impulse was no longer considered a valid reason to be considered NGRI. In addition, changes were made so that the defense now has to prove the defendant is insane, rather than the prosecution proving the defendant is sane. Consequently, the use of the NGRI defense is narrowed even further than in the past. In some states, there is a new verdict called "guilty but mentally ill."

ES   Moderate   Page: 591   kind: c

17.98: What are the two broad, philosophical rationales for the government's power to put people into psychiatric hospitals against their will, through civil commitment procedures?

Answer: Parens patriae: the government has a humanitarian responsibility to care for its weaker members. Police power: the government has a responsibility to protect society from danger.

ES   Moderate   Pages: 596-597   kind: c

17.99: A public policy official reads that the rates of violence are 5 times higher among patients with serious mental illness than among the general population. Based on this evidence, the public policy official recommends legislation that would allow patients with serious illness to be detained for longer periods than other people when arrested for minor offenses. What is the scientific evidence suggesting that such a policy is not justified?

Answer: 90% of the seriously mentally ill are never violent. A current psychotic episode is predictive of violence, but past psychotic episodes are not predictive of violence. Other factors besides mental illness also increase the risk for violence, such as poverty and drug use.

ES   Moderate   Page: 598   kind: c

17.100: Describe the 3 components of hospitalized patients' right to treatment, as established by the court case Wyatt v. Stickney in 1972.

Answer: A humane psychological and physical environment; quality staff in sufficient numbers; individualized treatment plans.

ES Difficult Page: 603 kind: c

17.101: How does Lenore Walker's concept of the battered woman syndrome explain why it is so hard for a battered women to leave an abusive relationship?

Answer: The cycle of violence in abusive relationships involves a period of loving contrition after episodes of abuse. Additionally, after repeated abuse, the abused person develops learned helplessness and passivity.

ES Moderate Page: 613 kind: c

17.102: Give at least one example of a case in which confidentiality must be broken by a therapist, and explain why confidentiality must be broken.

Answer: Suspected child abuse; when the patient is dangerous to self or others; when the patient has threatened to harm someone. Confidentiality must be broken in order to protect people's lives and to protect victims of child abuse.

ES Easy Page: 616 kind: c